TO CHA̶ ̶ ̶
WITH LOVE & RESPECT.
LEONARD

# YOUR
# CONSCIENCE

### The Key to Unlock
### Limitless Wisdom and Creativity
### and Solve All of Life's Challenges

FIRST EDITION

AMI Publishers
PO Box 430, Averill Park, New York 12018, Tel. (518) 674-8714
**amipublishers.org • info@amipublishers.org**

The American Meditation Institute, Inc.
Averill Park, New York, Tel. (518) 674-8714
**americanmeditation.org • ami@americanmeditation.org**

The paper used in this book meets the minimum requirements of the American National Standard for Information Sciences—Permanence of Paper for Printed Library Materials, ANSI Z39.48-1984.

Printed in the United States of America • Cover Design by George Foster

Cover illustration: Sashkin7 © 123RF.com; illustration on page 49 © 2021 American Meditation Institute; illustration on page 54 Yupiramos © 123RF.com; illustrations on pages 60 and 103 © American Meditation Institute; photograph on page 104 © 2004, Michael Dzamen Photography, Troy, New York; photographs on pages 135, 137, 138, 140, 142 © American Meditation Institute; photograph on page 141 Fizkes © 123RF.com; photograph on page 143 Rido © 123RF.com; photograph on page 144 Lightfield studios © 123RF.com.

Library of Congress Control Number: 2021905011
ISBN 9780975375266 (pbk. : alk. paper) I ISBN 9780975375259 (Ebook)

10 9 8 7 6 5 4 3 2  First Edition, 2021

# YOUR CONSCIENCE

The Key to Unlock
Limitless Wisdom and Creativity
and Solve All of Life's Challenges

FIRST EDITION

## LEONARD PERLMUTTER (RAM LEV)

**with Jenness Cortez Perlmutter**

**AMI Publishers**
Averill Park, New York 12018

## *Dedication*

We humbly dedicate this book to the Conscience—the divine capacity of the human mind to access unalloyed Truth in every moment, and to empower us to fulfill the purpose of our lives.

# A Call to Humanity

*Dare to know! Have the courage to use your own intelligence.*

IMMANUEL KANT

*A bit of advice given to a young Native American at the time of his
initiation: As you go the way of life, you will see a great chasm.
Jump! It's not as wide as you think.*

JOSEPH CAMPBELL

I wrote this book to address a crisis in education.

Many of us, no matter when we graduated from high
school, were only educated to memorize and recite information. Perhaps a truly skilled teacher taught us critical
thinking skills. *But it is highly unlikely that we learned to
develop the practical and creative tools that reliance on the
Conscience can provide.* As a result, we are ignorant of our
own innate, brilliant human capacity to make the wise and
kind decision in every circumstance. The Conscience gives
us the confidence to know what's to be done and what's
not to be done, no matter what challenge we face. But our
ignorance of the power of the Conscience blinds us and
leads to suffering.

The relentless onslaught of information from our mobile devices, cable news, emails, and social media feeds adds yet another layer of stress and anxiety we are not equipped to manage. At an alarming rate, bits of new data challenge our security and titillate the pleasure centers in our brains, driving us to make snap decisions that lead to fear, anger, disease and even death. Technology may have changed how we were taught and how we stay connected to one another, but it has not addressed this serious deficit in our collective education.

At this auspicious moment, an openness to embracing new (and old) ideas from beyond our present cultural matrix can bring us the sustenance and growth we desperately need and desire. Our modern American culture now faces a golden opportunity to go beyond its impoverished rigidity, superstition, blind customs and dogma to attain the spiritual and philosophical wealth necessary to solve *all* of life's challenges.

Today, a new reliance on our Conscience as our guide can make it possible for each of us to access and integrate intuitive wisdom, and to establish greater personal security, creativity and peace of mind. As we experiment with the profound gifts of the Conscience to determine our thoughts, words and deeds, we are destined to become both prophets and beneficiaries of our own Super Conscious Wisdom. For this noble endeavor, learning how to use the infinite resources of the Conscience is not simply a good idea, it is a dire necessity.

With love and respect,
Leonard Perlmutter (Ram Lev)

# Table of Contents

## RESOURCES

# *Acknowledgements*

We gratefully acknowledge the love and teachings of our first Gurus, our parents, Clara and Julius Perlmutter and Frances and Jesse Northerner, from whom we first learned about the Conscience.

We humbly offer our deep gratitude to our revered master, Shri Swami Rama of the Himalayas, and the countless women and men of the ancient Bharati spiritual lineage who have selflessly stewarded the priceless teaching of Yoga Science through millenia. In addition, we acknowledge the important influences of Eknath Easwaran, Swami Dayananda Saraswati, Nisargadatta Maharaj, and the teachings of Moses, Jesus the Christ, Krishna and the Compassionate Buddha.

We are very deeply grateful to Jennifer Masters, whose "big picture" vision, generosity and inspired editing have been essential in shaping this book. Thanks also to George and Mary Foster for their creative cover design.

We express our appreciation to our beloved secretary, Elaine Peterson, for the sharing of her many gifts that enable us to do our work in the world. And to Vikash Agrawal, Mary Balsam, Michelle Becker, Valerie Chakedis, Tom Doherty and the entire Cardinal Publishers Group,

Laurie Gold, DJ Hellerman, Suzanne Martin, George Mayer, Teri Mayor, Heather Rivenburg, André Tremblay and Sandy Vo, we offer our gratitude for their ongoing insights and support.

With respect and gratitude we also acknowledge the visionary work of the AMI Department of Medical Education: Co-Chair Renee Rodriguiz-Goodemote MD, Co-Chair Anthony Santilli MD, Chair Emeritus Beth Netter MD, Kristin Kaelber MD PhD, Anita Burock-Stotts MD, Jesse Ritvo MD, Donna Heffernan MD, Mark Pettus MD, Susan Lord MD, Bernie Siegel MD, Peggy Jacob RN, Gustavo Grodnitzky PhD and Mary Helen Holloway AMI-MT.

Last but not least, we are eternally grateful for the profound lessons taught to us by all the courageous seekers we have been priviledged to teach and to serve.

# *Special Notes*

### Italic Usage

Please note that Sanskrit words and names of concepts are printed in *italic* to enhance your familiarity with them.

### Capitalizations

Certain words are capitalized to denote that they refer to the Supreme Reality; the Supreme Intelligence.

### Pronunciation of Sanskrit Terms

To help you become more comfortable with these new words, please refer to this brief guide.

**Ahimsa** - ah him' suh
**Buddhi** - rhymes with hoodie
**Manas** - mahn' us
**Preya** - pray' uh
**Shreya** - shray' uh (rhymes with preya)

# *Introduction*

*A problem cannot be solved
on the level at which it appears.
It must be solved on a higher level.*

ALBERT EINSTEIN

We live in challenging times. Whether it is the affairs of the world or a more private struggle that disturbs your peace, solutions can feel elusive. Some days are better than others, of course, when kindness and grace and insight appear—like those brilliant shafts of light we see when the sun pierces a thick cloud. But some days are worse, when fear and anxiety overwhelm, and there is no light in sight, at least not in your corner of the world.

Each of us faces challenges every day, large and small: health, job stress, difficult family relationships, finances, education, violence, prejudice in all its hurtful forms, and more. As Einstein so wisely advised, we cannot solve these problems by relying on the same kind of thinking that got us into trouble in the first place. In other words, we must seek a higher knowledge. I know you are not Einstein—

neither am I—but *each one of us, including you, already has access to the source of the greater wisdom and creativity we need to solve life's most difficult challenges.* This book is meant to help you discover, assimilate and employ that wisdom.

Let's begin our exploration with an old, mythological story about the beginning of time. Long ago, when the universe was being created and everything was just about ready to go live, the Creator realized there was one final task to complete. So an angel was summoned.

When the angel arrived, the Supreme Intelligence—a.k.a. God, Adonai, Allah, Brahman, Divine Mother, Great Spirit—told the angel that there was one last job to do before the universe could be fully functional.

"I saved the best for last," the Creator told the angel. "In my hands I hold the key for accessing the highest wisdom, the power to creatively resolve all of life's challenges. This sacred treasure is of infinite value, and when it is finally found, human beings will know its blessings to be inexhaustible. We need to find a safe place to protect this treasure!"

So the angel agreed to the task and offered up an idea, "I will hide the treasure of life on top of the highest mountain peak."

"The treasure will be too easy to find there," replied the Creator.

"Okay," said the angel, "then I will hide your treasure in the middle of the largest and driest desert on planet Earth. Surely, they won't look there."

"Nope, too easy."

"In the vast reaches of the universe?" asked the angel. "That would definitely make for a demanding search."

"No," the Creator said, while contemplating. Then, in a flash of Supreme Genius these words were spoken: "I've got it! Hide the highest Wisdom of Life *within human beings.* They will look there last, and know how precious and valuable this treasure is. Yes, hide the treasure there."

This wisdom, and the search for it, are the subjects of sacred texts from every tradition—East and West. It is known by names such as: Holy Spirit, Soul, Divine Light, and Super Conscious Wisdom, to name just a few. The words we use to describe it are all inadequate! This wisdom is accessible to all, *but* given the predictable habit patterns of human beings, this treasure has indeed been well hidden. The last place we humans look for solutions is within ourselves. Instead, we look everywhere else—to religion and philosophy, technology, politics, art, education, sex, food, sleep, travel, consumerism, psychological therapies, a variety of addictive substances, this or that person, this or that hobby or profession. Yet again and again, with each well-meaning effort, we come away no better off than we were. We still have not found a reliable method of accessing and utilizing the highest wisdom to resolve life's issues—both simple and complex. And in the process, we deplete our energy and remain in pain.

Unfortunately, the real meaning and value of pain is not well understood. Pain presents invaluable guidance. In actuality, pain is the shadow of the outstretched hand of the Supreme Intelligence advising us that there is some form of friction in our lives. The friction exists between the limited perspectives of our undisciplined mind, and the Super Conscious Wisdom that is always available to lead us to greater awareness, creativity and reward.

We may have accepted pain as a familiar, unwelcome companion for years, but at a certain point we begin to recognize that if we always do what we've always done, we'll always get what we always got. That honest assessment prepares us to examine our lives, and to discover new possibilities that can bring us the purpose, freedom and happiness we deeply desire. Through that new clarity of vision, we arrive at a point of openness to change. Perhaps that time is now, for you.

Perhaps you are coping with a serious illness. Perhaps you've graduated from high school or college, and don't know what comes next. Maybe you just retired. Or maybe you have questions about gender or sexual orientation. Maybe you have been working for decades to realize "a more perfect union," and you are simply exhausted. Perhaps someone you love dearly has recently died. Perhaps you lost your job, and you're trying to figure out what you're meant to do in this world. Maybe you still have a job, but it's not rewarding. Or you don't have enough money to pay your bills, much less to buy the things that would make life more comfortable. Perhaps you can't sleep because you're habitually plagued by worry. Perhaps you have recently broken up with your partner, or perhaps your partner has recently broken up with you.

Maybe you feel like you are (mostly) doing fine, but you can't shake the feeling that something is just a little "off," that there's something missing, something more meaningful to be found in life.

Or perhaps, for no reason you can identify, you felt a little spark of curiosity when your eyes landed on this book, and rather than ignore it, you chose to pause and honor that little spark.

Whatever the reason, I am glad you are here. Our karmas have brought us together. There it is, that word: *karma*. We throw it around so freely, yet many of us don't understand its true meaning. The Law of Karma states, quite simply, that actions result in consequences. Or, as Sir Isaac Newton stated in his Third Law of Motion, every action gives rise to an equal reaction, or "fruit" of that action. Many of us learned this in school, and we see examples of it every day of our lives. We push on a door, and the door opens.

It is the *mechanics behind* the Law of Karma that make things interesting, however, and that is the subject of this book.

What do I mean by the mechanics behind the Law of Karma? I will answer with a question: What makes a human being—you, me, anybody—take an action? In other words, what initiates an action? Before I continue with my explanation, please take a moment to read that question again. Slow down, and contemplate your answer before you continue reading.

Consider this: before you or I take any particular action (in word or deed), we must first *entertain a thought*. Before we push on the door, we must *think* about pushing on the door. Sometimes we are consciously aware of the thought, for example, "I am angry." In response to that thought, I might act by walking away, yelling or slamming the door shut. Often, however, we are less aware of the thoughts that cause us to act, as when we do something unconsciously, simply because it is a longstanding habit. Either way, the thought comes first, and then the action. As it turns out, the mechanics behind of the Law of Karma are also uncompromising: *thought leads to action, and action leads to consequence.*

If we accept that every action begins with a thought, then the study of the mind—as the source of all thoughts—becomes the key to experiencing a lifetime of positive consequences. *Remember, consequences always have their beginnings in the mind.* We are the architects of our lives. We determine our destiny, and if we honor the Law of Karma with discrimination, our destiny can be a life of good health, abundance, and loving, nurturing relationships.

This examination of the Law of Karma, the power of thoughts, and their relationships with action and consequence, leads us logically to Yoga Science. Five to six thousand years ago, the pioneers of modern Yoga Science dealt with similar stressors in their own lives—how to keep themselves and their loved ones safe, how to find meaning and purpose in their lives, how to be healthy and happy. Instead of seeking solutions outside themselves, some women and men embarked on journeys of self-inquiry and self-discovery. By experimenting with the scientific principles of the Law of Karma, they learned how to unify the wisdom potential of the mind with the skillfully dynamic capacities of the body. Through their process of internal research and mental experimentation, these early Yoga Scientists received a priceless, practical Wisdom that can serve us well today—if we are motivated to follow in their footsteps. They figured out where that most precious treasure was hidden, and we can too.

Yoga Science provides a scientific "template" to access and employ the same higher knowledge that physicist, mathematician and mystic Albert Einstein spoke of. This same Wisdom is described in all the texts of our world's religious and spiritual traditions. It's a blueprint for experiencing happiness, health and security while fulfilling the purpose of life without pain, misery or enslavement. Sounds pretty attractive, right? It is.

In fact, Yoga Science, the world's oldest holistic mind/body medicine, offers us a hands-on framework for gathering, measuring and organizing data, making predictions, testing those predictions with repeatable experiments, and drawing conclusions. The conclusions derived from each Yoga Science experiment then become the basis for our daily thoughts, words and deeds. Gradually we learn to live in accord with the Law of Karma and to act more skillfully, lovingly and rewardingly in all realms of life—physical, mental, emotional and spiritual. The laboratory for every Yoga Science experiment is your very own mind-body-sense complex. No special equipment required.

So, that is where we will begin, each of us exactly where we are in our minds and bodies. If you are an earnest seeker, Yoga Science will offer you great benefits, regardless of your current level of experience, knowledge or state of mind.

Along the way, we will practice *ahimsa*. The word *ahimsa* means non-injuring, non-harming or non-violence. Sometimes it is translated as "kindness," and is simply a restatement of the Golden Rule: Do unto others as you would have others do unto you. It is the highest yogic principle and underlies every successful relationship— within and without, subtle and gross, with others *and with yourself*.

When learning a new frame of reference or a skill of any kind, we can sometimes become impatient with our lack of understanding or progress. I will remind you throughout our journey together to be kind to yourself as you study, assimilate and experiment with this teaching. This is a transformational process, and a life-long one at that. Have patience. Be kind to yourself. Practice *ahimsa*. To become proficient in any endeavor in life requires ongoing dedication. This is especially true with the study and practice of learning how the mind works. Because the Unconscious mind is filled with a field of unhelpful forces (for instance fear, anger and complacency) that can undercut your efforts, it is best to start by taking small steps. Don't take on too much too soon.

Start with what's easy, and the choice will be exactly right for you. In order to be the right choice, it must be easy. If you wanted to become a body builder, you wouldn't rush to the gym and, with no prior experience, attempt to bench-press two hundred pounds. You'd start by lifting just the bar with no additional weight. Then, you'd gradually add five pounds, then ten pounds, then twenty— until you reached your ultimate goal. I urge you to take the same reasonable (and kind!) approach as you begin to train your mind.

One final word on my experience with the wisdom presented in this book. My wife Jenness and I have studied and applied Yoga Science and philosophy for 55 years because this teaching is eminently practical and common-sensical. It has prepared us to make wise choices in every relationship and situation that arises. We have never disengaged from the world or our culture. Rather, we have lived our adult lives working, playing and facing the same challenges you face. Since 1971, Jenness has earned a living as a professional artist, and I as her art dealer—careers that we continue to enjoy today. As a consequence of our life-long commitment to practicing and experimenting with Yoga Science, in 1996 our teacher, Swami Rama of the Himalayas, directed us to "Start teaching now." In service to his instruction, we founded The American Meditation Institute in our home near Albany, New York. This was not the life either of us had imagined or desired, yet we were called to do this work and to share these teachings, and it has offered us unbounded happiness and fulfillment.

If you have ever gone to a yoga or a meditation class, you may have been greeted by your teacher with a smile and the word *Namaste*, which means "I honor the Supreme Intelligence in you." Even if you haven't had that experience, it's likely you've heard the word somewhere. Like that word *karma*, it seems to have worked its way into our collective vocabulary—even if we haven't yet fully grasped its meaning. I hope it will resonate more deeply for you by the time you finish this book. Thank you for being here. I am honored to be with you. *Namaste*.

# *Conscience*

kon'-shəns

The English word "Conscience" is derived from the Latin preposition *con*, meaning with, and the infinitive *scire*, to know. "With knowledge." "With wisdom." "With science."

*Scire* also means to make bright; to cause to shine by reflected light; to be effulgent in splendor or beauty; to be eminent, conspicuous, or distinguished; to exhibit brilliant intellectual powers; to be immediately apparent; to distinguish oneself; to excel; to emit or reflect light.

From this luminous word *scire* comes the word *scio*, which means I know. I understand. I have knowledge. *I emit brilliance, splendor, beauty and light.*

It is the job of our Conscience to reflect that brilliance, that confidence, that unerring wisdom, as we go about our lives determining the best course of action—what to do, and what not to do—in every circumstance, with every relationship. It is the aim of this book to present ancient teachings that will guide you in that daily process. I am confident that what you are about to read will feel instantly and intimately familiar to you.

Let's begin.

CHAPTER 1

# *In Pleasure and Pain, Victory and Defeat: Who am I?*

*All that a Guru can tell you is:*
*'Dear One, you are quite mistaken about yourself.*
*You are not the person you take yourself to be.'*

NISARGADATTA MAHARAJ

Our aim is to understand the mind so we can more skillfully resolve life's many challenges. And there are plenty of them. We each face individual and societal challenges every day, regardless of our age, gender, educational background, profession, political ideology, race, class, or any other label that might be used to describe us.

If you objectively examine your own world, you'll notice that the core issue in every challenge you face centers on change—either your attraction to it, or your rejection of it. Today's technological wizardry compresses the rate of change from decades, centuries or millennia to weeks, days, hours—even minutes. Other times, the pace of change seems so slow that we notice no movement at all.

Change can be perceived as bad or good, but regardless of how you view it, in some way change always represents a death. I am not talking only about the death of a person. Change can mean the death of a friendship, a job, an outdated policy or your first gray hair. Change happens all the time, everywhere. Certainly we must deal with occasional traumatic change like serious illness, the death of a loved one, or the sudden loss of financial security. But these traumatic changes are not everyday occurences. Rather, it's the relentless rate and volume of daily change that is the problem. Change is served up in a never-ending loop through our 24-hour news cycle and social media feeds. We simply never get a break from change and its partner, fear.

We are regularly triggered by news stories and images that leave uncertainty, stress, anxiety and exhaustion in their wake. As a result, the reptilian portion of our brain never deactivates the fight-flight-freeze response that warns us of potential danger. We remain in a perpetual state of high alert, and our mind tends to catastrophize. We focus on the small rather than the big picture. We resist change and look for someone to blame for our pain. In a state of confusion, the mind retreats to what's familiar, preventing us from examining the truth of our situation and adding to our insecurity and fear. Meanwhile, our body is being poisoned by a cascade of stress hormones. All in all, not a good prescription for a happy, healthy, rewarding life.

For most of us, the cumulative weight of these factors can feel crushing. But this state of dis-ease also begs the question, "Is there anything I can do right now to end the gnawing fear, anger, depression and the feeling that things are out of control?"

The short answer is YES! But only if you're willing to examine, and then say goodbye to some old, unhelpful, and astonishingly stubborn habits of the mind. If you're ready for a new perspective on your own mind, let's begin our journey together.

At this point in history, two opposing forces are vying for our attention. The first (akin to the "Big Bang" theory of physics) is an externally-oriented drive that motivates us to seek happiness and security in the endless procession of objects and relationships that come from outside of us. The second force is the opposite. It's an inwardly-directed drive that motivates us to seek, find and employ the hidden treasure of wisdom and creativity at the core of our being.

Right from the start, you need to understand that the kind of effort required to choose the inward path is not always easy—in part because self-reliance is neither fashionable nor valued in today's world. To grow and sustain your own self-reliance, you must be willing to resist the cultural suggestion that you can rely exclusively on others for your happiness. At best, outside suggestions are hearsay, and therefore never completely reliable. That's why William Shakespeare reports his experience with the truth by advising, "Above all else, to thine own Self be true."

But be careful! What did Shakespeare mean by "thine own Self?" He was not just talking about your intellectual mind, no matter how keen it might be. In the next chapter we will explore in depth the Four Functions of the Mind identified by the ancient sages of Yoga Science. For now, suffice it to say that even the most brilliant logic is not enough to resolve life's seemingly unresolvable challenges. Intellectual knowledge, however attractive and well intentioned it may be, has little power to change character, conduct or consciousness. Your Conscience is the only function of the mind that can reliably unlock your Super Conscious Wisdom, enabling you to transform the powerful, poisonous energy of negative emotions into previously unimagined, creative and rewarding solutions. We will talk much more about this.

In actuality, your painful circumstances today reflect a deep-seated struggle between the forces of darkness and light within your own individual mind. Yes, the mind is your problem, *but the mind is also your solution*. While your past actions are forcing you to engage in this battle within, you must first decide on which side you will fight. This book was written to help you make this crucial decision. Remember, you are the architect of your life, and you determine your destiny—by what you trust in, think about, speak of, and act on. All of this begins within your own mind.

Here's a concept that might be helpful. *Eucatastrophe* is a word coined around 1937 by J. R. R. Tolkien, author of *Lord of the Rings*. The term refers to a sudden and apparently disastrous turn of events which, despite initial appearances, results in the hero or heroine's salvation. Best of all, this stunningly positive resolution comes not from some outside intervention, but from within the existing elements of the disaster. Tolkien formed the word by adding the Greek prefix *eu*, meaning good, to the word *catastrophe*, meaning momentous misfortune. The implications are profound and practical and in perfect harmony with the teaching presented in this book.

Tolkien has given a name to an important, yet often doubted truth: even events that at first seem unacceptable always hold the potential for benefit. If we accept this truth, we are emboldened to transform negativity into creativity. But how? As we strive to make the best choices in the face of the numerous challenges we must acknowledge that *the unexamined and unconscious preconceptions of our minds will exert enormous power to distort our perception.*

Without the ability to see situations clearly, creative solutions to life's challenges will continue to elude us.

These very same unconscious preconceptions will also impact the seemingly mundane choices we make each day—what to have for dinner, what to read or watch on TV, when to go to bed. Old habit patterns are particularly effective at temporarily reducing our capacity for clarity.

Our task is to learn to skillfully manage our mind in order to restore that clarity—the Super Conscious Wisdom that will guide us in what to think, what to say, and what to do. But what does it look like, that Wisdom? That precious treasure? It looks like You. Your truest and best Self. That is the subject of this chapter. After 26 years of teaching and 55 years of study, I have found it helpful to begin with the end in mind, to agree upon a shared goal. So I offer here a description of the treasure, your highest Self— that is, Self with a capital "S." Chances are, it is not what you think.

In everyday life none of us really sees circumstances as they truly are. Instead, we experience a projection of our own mental concepts. As first century Greek philosopher Epictetus said, "We are not disturbed by things, but rather by the views we hold of them." Shakespeare went so far as to claim that, "There is nothing either good or bad, but thinking makes it so."

Because so many of our unconsciously held concepts are neither true nor valid, the perceptions our minds form, and the associated actions our bodies take, often lead to more pain—not the desired overcoming of pain. If we seek solutions while relying on worn-out, untruthful, faulty concepts, we will doom ourselves to even more pain. Unintentionally, we will create yet another level of distress. As the Compassionate Buddha warned, "Don't swallow a hot iron ball and then cry out, 'I am in great pain.'"

If we are sincerely seeking a kinder and more reward-ing way to treat ourselves and others (remember *ahimsa*, the highest principle of Yoga Science—non-injury, non-harming), we must first examine the one concept that most perverts our human perceptions. That concept is the per-sonal pronoun "I."

Sadly, in the midst of all our human relationships, most of us do not really know who we are. Some of us spend years trying to figure it out on our own. Others more will-ingly accept the judgments of our families, friends, thera-pists, doctors, colleagues, even our spiritual leaders. But if those "advisors," regardless of how well-meaning they may be, seek to know us merely by evaluating our current physical, mental, emotional, political and spiritual attrib-utes, they can never really know us for certain. Why? Because everything with a name and a form in the material world is continually changing—including "me," and in-cluding "you."

This state of continual change means that in the material world where we live, everything is relative. As we already know, Einstein intuitively advised us that "A problem cannot be solved on the level at which it appears. It must be solved on a higher level." If we can admit to ourselves that we need to set aside all *relative truth* in order to find meaningful solutions to life's challenges, we will be well on our way to ending suffering and ushering joy into all our relationships.

But what do I mean by setting aside relative truth? How is this done? The first step to discovering the higher Truth that Einstein believed would lead to genuine and workable solutions, is to contemplate and answer this essential question: Who am I? We must spend some time stripping away our misconceptions about ourselves and get back to basics.

## Who am I?

We define ourselves physically, mentally, emotionally and spiritually every day. We might define ourselves as tall or short, heavy or thin, flexible or inflexible, happy or sad, focused or unfocused, calm or stressed, angry or forgiving, bored or interested, fearful or fearless. The list could go on and on.

When we examine how we define ourselves, one thing becomes clear. Each definition of "I" implies the existence of its polar opposite. Why? Because our world of relativity is defined by pairs of opposites. We can't know up without knowing down, in without knowing out, anger without knowing forgiveness, and fearlessness without knowing fear.

If you gaze at the ceiling above you it will appear high to you, and yet if you were on the roof, that same ceiling would seem low. While that observation would also be true, both would be only *relatively* true. On this plane of existence that we call our daily lives, the human being is also subject to the laws of relativity. The height of the ceiling, for example, is subject to the laws of time, space and causation. The ceiling height is only relatively true, *and relative truths are always subject to change.*

The very same can be said about any definition we attribute to the personal pronoun "I." Information derived through the Senses (what we see, taste, hear, smell, or feel) is always only relatively true. Right now I'm tall, but when I was five years old I was short. Yesterday I was angry, but today I'm forgiving. Last week I was calm, yet this week I'm anxious. When I fly in an airplane twenty thousand feet in the air, I am fearful. When the plane lands I become fearless. On the first day of class, I was confused. Now I understand a new concept, and I feel smarter.

Is there *anything* that is not relative, you might ask.

Anything that does not change? The ancient sages tell us there is but one constant: *the only unchanging truth about ourselves that we can declare with certainty is "I AM."* Other than I AM, when we try to define ourselves we invariably settle on a meaning that reflects a relative truth that is ever-changeable. Everyday definitions of the "I" are never absolutely true.

Let's pause for a moment and contemplate this point. Based on your memory, was there ever a time in your life when the statement "I am" was not absolutely true?

Certainly the size and shape of your body have changed over a lifetime, as has your mental and emotional landscape. You might have been heavy as a child, but now you are thin. Yesterday you might have been ill, but today you're healthy. In your youth you were politically liberal, but in the afternoon of life you're more conservative, or the other way around.

The "I-am-ness" that has continued as the only constant in your life is the most persuasive indication that an unchanging consciousness exists beyond the mind-body-sense complex that "I" refer to as "me." *That consciousness, the "I-am-ness," has never ceased to be, no matter what changes around it.* This inherent capacity to be present every moment—to witness—is what allows "you" to perceive and comprehend the words on this page, and it enables "me" to order thoughts and create this book.

### Consciousness and the Objects of Consciousness

Consciousness, sometimes referred to as awareness, exists both within and beyond time, with and without an object to observe. When we learn to observe our thoughts, the consciousness within us can observe the consciousness that exists even in the silence between two thoughts. Consciousness is the background of all reality—a cosmic soup of awareness from which and into which all gross and subtle objects appear for limited periods of time. Maybe that sounds a little too "esoteric" and "deep"to you. But stay with me, and stay open. An understanding of this ever-present inner consciousness and the nature of the objects it can observe will serve you well.

What are these gross and subtle objects that continually appear in your awareness? The clothes you wear and the bed you sleep in are gross objects. Anything that's perceived through the Senses is a gross object—including the human body. The truth, therefore, is that "we" have a body, and "we" are *aware* of the body, but "we" are *not* the body. Our body and brain are merely the instruments of consciousness.

Gross objects appear in your awareness for only a limited time, and then they depart. Gross objects, in addition to our own bodies, include all the people and things we come into contact with every day. This phenomenon is not very different from the weather. Yesterday it was sunny. Today it's raining, and tomorrow it may snow. None of these gross objects is permanent. Each one is always in flux.

Subtle objects also appear in your awareness for only a limited time. Subtle objects include thoughts, desires, emotions and concepts that appear, and then disappear from your consciousness. Like gross objects, subtle objects also have a form, but they vibrate at a frequency too high to be perceived through the rudimentary instrumentation of the five Senses. You can't see, taste, or touch them. Yet, through the mind, your most powerful instrument, "you" (the consciousness within you, that *is* you) are made aware of these subtle objects. Seemingly out of nowhere, a thought comes into your awareness. It could be a thought that provokes a desire, fear or anger. It might not have been in your awareness a few seconds ago, yet you're aware of it now, in the present moment. In an hour you may hardly remember the thought. Subtle objects are always changing. And the many thousands of thoughts you have every day are among those subtle objects.

This understanding encourages us to dis-identify with anything that is transitory. It is clear "you" have a body, but "you" are not the body. "You" have a mind with thoughts, desires, emotions and concepts, but "you" are not the mind, nor are "you" the thoughts, desires, emotions or concepts appearing in your awareness through the instrument of the mind. *Essentially, the real You is awareness itself.* The *real* You is pure consciousness without any object—consciousness that, by its very nature, can perceive all the gross and subtle objects that appear in time and space. "You" can never completely define who "You" are through the limitations of language, but "You" can experience the Truth. Is there anything that can be said, then, about the nature of the *real* You? Yes. Yoga Science uses three Sanskrit words to describe our Essential Nature as a composition of three fundamental qualities—*Sat, Chit* and *Ananda.*

### *Sat*—Eternal Existence

The first characteristic of your Essential Nature (the *real* "I") is described by the Sanskrit word *Sat,* meaning eternal existence. The internal witnessing capacity that allows "you" to perceive all gross and subtle objects is eternal and changeless. The ultimate "I" was never born and will never die. It is self-existent. Unlike every gross and subtle object, awareness is not dependent on anything else for its existence.

No object can claim to be eternal. This book, for example, is neither eternal nor self-existent. It is dependent on many different things for its existence: trees, a lumberjack, trucker, paper mill, printer, bindery, author, editor, publisher, salesperson, and bookstore or website. Objects like a book, or even the desire for the knowledge to make an enlightened decision about any small or large challenge you face, may be subject to change, but your own awareness—which empowers perception—is eternal.

Let's look at what the Bible says about our eternal nature. (If you have an allergic reaction to this particular text, please try to set your preconceptions aside, and read on.) Jesus the Christ taught us that, "Before Abraham was, I am." What was He speaking of, if not the eternal capacity to witness? When Moses was in the desert, he stood before a bush that was burning yet not consumed by the flames. Acknowledging the sacredness of the experience, Moses asked the bush, "Who are you?" Whereupon the bush replied to Moses, "I am that I am." Moses grasped this Divine pronouncement, but he still was doubtful that others would. He asked the bush, "What shall I tell the Hebrew people? Who shall I tell them has sent me?" To this the Supreme Intelligence responded by saying, "Tell the Hebrew people that 'I am' has sent you." When placed in the context of Yoga Science, the true meaning of these verses begins to open up for us.

### *Chit* – Consciousness and Wisdom

The second characteristic of your Essential Nature ("I") is *Chit*, meaning consciousness—your capacity for awareness, attention and wisdom. *Within consciousness resides an intuitive library of wisdom* known as the Super Conscious Mind. This is the Wisdom hidden at the core of your being, that precious buried treasure you can unlock by coordinating the Four Functions of the Mind (described in the next chapter) and heeding the voice of your own Conscience. Your Super Conscious Wisdom is the source of Truth, love, and creativity.

Every day, you have relationships with thousands of

gross objects: people, animals, plants and minerals. You also witness thousands of subtle objects: thoughts, desires, emotions and judgments that come into your awareness for a limited length of time. The nature of the *real* "I" is Eternal Awareness, or Eternal Consciousness (*Sat* and *Chit*)—capable of providing all the higher knowledge necessary to solve the seemingly unsolvable, and to fulfill your life's purpose.

### *Ananda* – Bliss or Fullness

The final characteristic of your Essential Nature ("I") is *Ananda*. This is the quality we are all seeking—and the truth is we already have it! *Ananda* means bliss or complete fullness. There is no gross or subtle object you can know, experience or obtain that can make you any fuller or more content than the pure consciousness, at the center of your being, already is. On the highest level of consciousness, "I" am the Eternal Witness—eternally content in the bliss and fullness of transcendent perfection.

You have already glimpsed this unspeakable joy, bliss, fullness and contentment that the sages refer to as *Ananda*, and yet, you may not have recognized it. You might have experienced this joy when you fell in love, or at the sight of your own newborn child. It may have come when you held your first puppy or kitten. Or, the bliss of *Ananda* might have briefly visited you as you jogged, gardened or read; as you lost yourself in a beautiful painting, musical composition or intimate sexual relationship; or as you stood in awe before the majesty of a glorious sunset on a secluded mountain lake. Some of you experienced a spiritual moment of fullness as a child or adolescent, but you did not possess the language to describe your experience to anybody. Still, you *know* it happened, and you have never forgotten the moment or the feeling. That is *Ananda*.

When your attention is completely captured by one

object, there is no room for thinking. You neither entertain memories of the past nor imaginations of the future. Instead, at that singular point in space and time, when all your attention becomes fixed on a particular object, the perceiver and the object of perception both disappear, and what reflects into the awareness of the Inner Witness is *Ananda*—an indescribable contentment.

After a short time, of course, new, compelling thoughts stream into your awareness. New, subtle objects appear, diverting the personality from the bliss of one-pointed attention, and you once again begin to think and question. You may have been momentarily absorbed in the absolute beauty of a rose, but the mind eventually intervenes by entertaining a thought. For instance, "Is this rose as magnificent as the one I grew last summer? It's awful hot. I'm thirsty. I'll have a cold drink." The intellect diffuses your focus and the bliss fades from conscious awareness. Once more you are swept away into the unending procession of memories of the past and hypotheticals for the future.

Those fleeting, bliss-filled moments might be termed "peek" experiences. Through them, you have been granted a tiny glimpse, a peek into the joy that is your very own Divine Nature. When your attention is thoroughly one-pointed, the individual self, the little Ego, that limited sense of "I" disappears, leaving only *Sat-Chit-Ananda*, the eternal, bliss-filled consciousness and wisdom of the Eternal Witness. I Am.

## Your Perfect Higher Self

When the mind experiences a moment of one-pointedness, the habitual march of mental distractions temporarily halts. In that stillness you feel wonderful. This contentment is nothing other than the bliss of *Ananda* reflecting into your own consciousness (*Chit*). It is your eternal Self (*Sat*). It is fullness. It is perfection. No object or relationship could make you feel any more content than you already are in that stillness.

These experiences of fullness are a taste of what is your birthright. There is nothing "you" have to get from outside yourself to be free of anger, judgment, fear, anxiety, stress, burnout, phobias, sorrow, spiritual longing, or any kind of physical, mental or emotional suffering. You merely have to recognize That which you are. When a sculptor stands before a raw block of marble, she might have a vision of an elephant. As she takes hammer and chisel in hand, she proceeds to remove everything from the block that is not elephant—until all that remains is the elephant.

It is the same for each one of us. When we chip away at the transitory characteristics we use to define ourselves (student, teacher, sister, mother, father, son, husband, wife, intellectual, carpenter, activist, entrepreneur, physician, nurse, friend, lover, and so on) we are left with what is Real. We are left with our true Self. We can respond to the question "Who am I?" with a new kind of answer, one based not on relative truths, but on the Eternal Truth. I am. *Sat-Chit-Ananda.*

From here, we are better equipped to find solutions. There is really no magic in your making discriminating and rewarding choices—regardless of whether you're deciding on what to have for breakfast, how to respond to your angry friend or neighbor, or how our society should deal with racism and other intractable issues. In the past, "you" didn't know your real Self, and your own unconscious concepts habitually motivated "you" to make choices that gave rise to pain, misery and enslavement. As 20th century mystic Ramana Maharshi observed, "The mind is consciousness which has put on limitations. The *real* You is originally unlimited and perfect. Later, You put on limitations and then identify with the mind's constraints." Let us find our way back to the unlimited and perfect, which will provide us relief in our world of assumed limitations.

As you become more familiar with these concepts through your own personal experience, your personality will begin to acknowledge your real Self as *Sat-Chit-Ananda*—eternal, consciousness, wisdom and bliss. The real You will begin to see things as they are, not as they once appeared. Then, through an ongoing dynamic process of experimentation, purification and transformation, the old personality's unconscious limitations will slowly fall away. The old "you" will become the *real* You, supported by a clarity of vision that enables "you" to serve as the creative and compassionate instrument of change you long to be.

We will build on this concept of the true Self, the *real* You, throughout the rest of this book. In the last two chapters, I will offer some simple experiments for you to try. Do not forget *ahimsa*! I do *not* suggest that you begin a 30-minute meditation practice tomorrow morning. You might not yet have the knowledge or skills to proceed with that course of action. So for now, we will start small. But we will start. As you identify less with the body, with the personality's everyday web of entanglements, judgments, comparisons, and likes and dislikes, your capacity to stay grounded in your Eternal Witness will become more familiar and more comfortable.

Let us now take a closer look at the mind, as a means to illuminate your Essential Nature—the *real* You—eternal, consciousness, wisdom, and bliss. An objective and scientific understanding of the Four Functions of the Mind will prepare you to undertake some simple experiments that will lead you to your own inner light, your Super

Conscious Wisdom—to that precious hidden treasure that is already within you, waiting to be discovered, and bursting forth with the joy *and the solutions* that you seek.

CHAPTER 2

# The Four Functions of the Mind

*We lie in the lap of immense intelligence,*
*which makes us receivers of its truth and organs of its activity.*
*When we discern justice, when we discern truth, we do*
*nothing by ourselves, but allow a passage to its beams.*

RALPH WALDO EMERSON

What is the mind? In ordinary usage, we employ the word several different ways. It can refer to the conscious utilization of our attention, as in "mindfulness," or "mind your manners." And it can also mean decision, resolve or intention, as in "make up your mind," or "I've got half a mind to go for a walk." Sometimes it's even used as a synonym for "brain," that indispensable physical organ that occupies your skull. In addition, the word "mind" commonly represents the sum of our thoughts—all those ceaseless interior dialogues that constitute our basic sense of "me" and the nature of "my" reality, as well as our capacity for every level of problem solving and relating.

This fuzziness of definition is arguably symptomatic of our culture's abiding discomfort with the idea of pinning down exactly what's going on in our heads. Perhaps it's an uneasiness with the unknown force that seems to be running the show, and the resulting suspicion that to examine the origins and implications of our thoughts too closely might in some way be dangerous. Maybe we've simply embraced the unfortunate conviction that our own amateur attempts to understand it all could not possibly be successful. We may indeed be aware that different "voices" are interacting through our thoughts, yet to distinguish, identify and evaluate them may seem to be a confusing task we're not prepared to undertake.

That reluctance is understandable. But the science of Yoga offers a simple, reliable and exceedingly useful template to demystify and manage the previously unmanageable and wayward mind.

The mind is our most powerful instrument. In 200AD, the Indian sage Patanjali codified the ancient oral tradition of Yoga Science into a coherent text known as the *Yoga Sutras*. In the first pronouncement of that scripture, Patanjali stated that "All yoga begins with an understanding and coordination of the functions of the mind." This does not mean suppression of the thought process, but rather, regulation and mastery of the mind. The human mind has the capacity to transform our deepest desires into the realities of the world we experience. A disciplined mind can be our best friend and strongest ally in that endeavor, and conversely, an undisciplined mind can be our fiercest adversary.

As explained in the Introduction, the Law of Karma states that every time we take an action, a consequence results. Further, every action must first be preceded by a thought. We cannot even raise our hand or speak a word before we entertain a thought. It is our mind that will direct our hand to rise, or our mouth and vocal cords to speak. Thought always precedes action, even if we are not consciously aware of that mental process. Once we appreciate the power of this essential relationship between our thoughts, our actions, and the resulting consequences, the nature of our decision-making emerges as a critical factor in determining our condition in this life. And where do we make our decisions? In our minds.

To explore the deepest aspects of our internal being and to deal successfully with the countless challenges we face in the external world, we must study all aspects of our mind. A firm grasp of the mind's four unique operations prepares us to establish coordination of these functions. Without inner coordination, serious conflicts eventually arise in the mind and will inevitably manifest as stress, burnout, pain and disease, all of which are obstacles to seeing viable, creative solutions to life's many challenges.

We become free of interior conflict by learning how to "parent" the mind. We need to quell the mind's "sibling rivalries" and encourage teamwork. In this chapter, we will learn to recognize and respect the unique characteristics and contributions of each of the Four Functions of the Mind before we can successfully coach them. A practical understanding of these four players helps us transform the latent power of thoughts, desires, emotions and concepts, thereby establishing relative calm in the mind. When we have successfully parented our mind, it becomes still, and we become aware of our Essential Nature, the eternal consciousness that is our Super Conscious Wisdom. In this state it is possible to live free from conflict and pain.

Through practice a Yoga Scientist learns to consciously evaluate the character and merit of each thought as it appears in their awareness. Probing questions emerge: what is the purpose of this thought, and what will be its consequence? To whom is this thought appearing? Who am I? Who is the thinker of the thought? All these questions cultivate identification with the Inner Witness: *Sat-Chit-Ananda*. From this higher perspective we can evaluate fairly the worthiness of each thought. It sounds like a lot of work at first, but with practice it becomes second nature, similar to the process of learning how to ride a bicycle. We feel unsure or intimidated when we get on the bike the first time, but we quickly learn how to use the handle bars and pedals to stay balanced and propel ourselves forward. Soon we have mastered a global skill that offers the potential for freedom and a great deal of joy.

We will draw upon the teachings of the Himalayan masters as we seek to understand the mind and the origins of our thoughts. The diagram on page 49 illustrates a wheel comprised of three basic components: the rim of the wheel, the spokes and the hub. The hub facilitates the turning of the spokes, and the rim of the wheel rotates as a result.

In this analogy, the rim of the wheel represents the human body and the actions we take every day. No movement can occur in the body unless and until there is movement somewhere in the Four Functions of the Mind. These functions of the mind are like the spokes of the wheel. The mind always moves first and the body follows.

The hub of this wheel is your Super Conscious Wisdom, the precious hidden treasure. It is your Eternal Witness (*Sat-Chit-Ananda*). The hub powers the mind, and the mind ultimately animates the body. Without the existence of the hub there could be neither mind nor body.

The four spokes in our analogy represent the four major functions of the mind:

**1. Logic and Five Senses   2. Ego
3. Unconscious Mind   4. Conscience**

## Logic and Five Senses (*Manas*)

Our capacity for logic and our five Senses work together as the primary information-gathering mechanism of the mind. In addition, this function of the mind continually asks the questions: "Should I do it?" or "Should I not do it?" In Sanskrit, this function is called *Manas*, which means mind, and it most closely aligns with what we Westerners consider our logical mind. *Manas* (Logic and Senses) operates both internally and externally; it is an importer and exporter of information.

As we move through life, relating to each thought, desire and emotion we experience, we continually face the decision of whether or not to take an action. Toward that end, the *Manas* collects various bits of pertinent information from the external and internal worlds. In order to gather information from the external world, *Manas* employs our five Senses and sense organs: sight (eyes), smell (nose), hearing (ears), taste (mouth) and touch (hands, feet and skin). These employees go out into the material world and bring back information about the multitude of objects with which we might engage in a relationship.

Think about the process of deciding if you will try something new, like going for a walk in an unfamiliar town. If you are already in that town, you will use your eyes and ears to gather information about the environment around you. If you are not there, you might ask a friend if she has ever been to that town and if she has any helpful information. Or you could read a book or turn to Google for recommendations. This is the *Manas* at work—going outward to collect all the information necessary so you can decide whether or not you will go for that walk. *Manas* also goes inward to consult the Ego and Unconscious mind to gather even more information. It is important to remember that the *Manas* performs this function and organizes the data, but it does not make the decision.

## Ego

We are all familiar with Western psychology's concept of the Ego, with its negative implications of exaggerated self-importance. But I offer the ancient, more broad definition that Yoga Science assigns to this function of the mind. In this framework, the Ego is concerned with only one thing: self-preservation. And it starts its work *very* early.

At your birth, in the midst of a disorienting assault of sensory stimulation, your innate desire for self-preservation propels you to search for comfort, safety and contentment. Above all else, you must live! You must learn quickly to eliminate the pain you experience as an infant, suddenly cast out from the comfort and safety of the womb. But how? You wave your arms and legs and cry out, but beyond that, you are helpless. Then, mercifully, you are introduced to someone who holds you and feeds you. All of your attention focuses down to a single point: the source of your comfort and well-being, your mother's breast (or the bottle your caregiver is holding for you).

You quiet down and become content as you experience a cessation of pain and the establishment of pleasure. You are aware of relative calm. You feel safe, secure, warm, nurtured, and loved. In the midst of this new pleasant experience, you reach your first profound, mistaken conclusions: "I am a separate entity. Mama is a separate entity, and certain objects and relationships in the world can bring me happiness and relieve my pain." In this moment, you see yourself as a subject, and everything else as an object. Where there had just been one, now there are two.

For most of us, this primary faulty conclusion (certainly understandable, given the circumstances!) will drive the Ego and shape our attitudes and behavior for the rest of our lives. The security of Mama's breast is replaced by an endless succession of different objects: a pacifier, a stuffed animal, a new outfit, a good grade, a high school diploma, a boyfriend, a girlfriend, an automobile, a college degree, a job, a house, a partner—even your own baby.

Yoga Science teaches that as we grow and mature, the Ego is the function of the mind that perceives every object or relationship as either pleasant or unpleasant, "good" or "bad." These judgments come naturally, because the Ego's only purpose is assuring self-preservation. As children grow, they become more and more susceptible to the cultural suggestions of advertising and other external "experts," which are designed to convince the Ego that a particular product or person or philosophy will alleviate pain or provide pleasure. By the time we are adults, our Egos are often running the show.

But in the Yoga Science framework, the Ego is just another source of data and information for the *Manas* (our Senses and logical mind). Information from the Ego can be valid and useful, but its inherent bias must be taken into account. The Ego can be quite persuasive indeed. It has years of practice being the loudest voice in the room— just think about the power of a crying baby.

We are typically (but not always) consciously aware of the input we receive from the first two functions of the mind, the Senses and Ego. *However, these two functions constitute only a very small portion of the totality of our mind.*

### Unconscious Mind (Memories and Habits)

For most of our lives, we remain unaware of the largest portion of our mind. The Unconscious mind is a reservoir of all our memories and habits, a storehouse of information defined as useful in fulfilling our desires. It is like a catalog of all pleasant and unpleasant memories, imaginations for the future, and the information and concepts we believe (often mistakenly) that we need for self-preservation. Our Unconscious mind also serves as the repository for fear, anger and unfulfilled desires.

The character of the Unconscious mind is analogous to wet sand. Just as a child easily creates channels of water in wet sand on a beach, we easily create impressions in our Unconscious mind. We do this by repeatedly giving our attention to any subtle object like a thought, desire, or emotion. In doing so, we create an indentation in the topography of our Unconscious mind—a little channel in the wet sand. As we give continued attention to the thought, desire or emotion, the channel that is formed becomes deeper, making it easier for our awareness to flow through it. Some channels are the result of healthy and creative thoughts, but other channels may result from habitual destructive or unhealthy thoughts. Either way, they are the pathways through which our consciousness habitually flows—and for much of our lives, we don't even realize that these influential pathways exist.

In its never ending quest for information, the *Manas* adds information retrieved from the internal world of the Unconscious mind, all those impressions in the sand, to the various suggestions of the Ego and the Senses. Remember, *Manas* exists solely to gather data. It does not have the capacity to make any decisions.

### *Manas* (Senses and Logic) Presents its Findings

When the *Manas* has finished its preliminary fact-finding, it presents its findings for consideration. Addressing our awareness, the *Manas* begins by saying, "You have two basic alternatives. There is alternative A, which will probably result in consequences one, two, and three, and there is alternative B, which will probably result in consequences four, five, and six. What is your decision? In support of which alternative will you take an action?"

## The Four Functions of the Mind

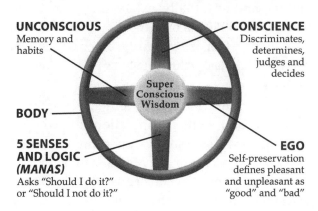

To explain the workings of the human mind, Yoga Science presents a simple, conceptual diagram: a wheel with four spokes that turn it. The rim of the wheel represents the body, and its hub is the Divine Super Conscious Wisdom that is our deepest nature. The four spokes represent the Four Functions of the Mind: **Senses and Logic** (Manas), **Ego** (self preservation), **Unconscious** (habits and memories), and **Conscience** (Buddhi). Ideally, these four functions work together in formulating every decision, large and small; but it is the Conscience that needs to have the last word if we are to live well and generously. In fact, it's the Conscience that makes every decision (the other functions don't have this capacity). But when the Senses, Ego, and Unconscious mind are clamoring loudly for attention, the contribution from the Conscience—offered in a steady, quieter voice—may be overlooked or overwhelmed. As a result, decisions may be made on the basis of incomplete or biased information.

After the *Manas* concludes its monologue on alternatives and consequences, it waits a bit for our decision. If none is forthcoming, it automatically begins again. "You have two basic choices: alternative A with certain consequences and alternative B with these different consequences. Have you made a decision yet?"

Without a decision, *Manas* repeats again and again, "You have two choices: A or B. Will you do it or will you not do it? What is your choice? A or B? A or B!? A or B!?!"

The relentless repetition first becomes annoying, then frustrating, and eventually, exhausting. The doubt and indecision play on like a broken record, and our inability or unwillingness to make a decision based on the available information is a major cause of stress in our lives.

In this respect, the functioning of *Manas* is analogous to the performance of the computer. No matter how sophisticated and swift its operation, the computer is always dealing with the solitary question: yes or no? (one or zero?). The function of the *Manas* is vital, but like the computer, it does not have the capacity to evaluate or to judge responsibly the information it collects and presents.

### Conscience (*Buddhi*)

The Conscience is the only function of the mind that has the ability to weigh the options and make a decision. In Sanskrit, this function is called the *Buddhi*, and its proper pronunciation rhymes with "hoodie." The *Buddhi* has the potential for great wisdom—a far greater wisdom than what today's cultural concepts ordinarily ascribe to the Conscience. It is much more than the little angel on your shoulder reminding you to eat your broccoli. (Although our Conscience can certainly help to make food choices that support the body.) *In fact, when the Conscience is functioning well, it reflects into our conscious mind that hidden treasure, the Super Conscious Wisdom that is buried deep inside each of us.* When employed regularly, the purified Conscience will have the reflective quality of a well-polished mirror, and can instantaneously access the infinite creativity, wisdom and love of the Supreme Intelligence at the center of consciousness.

This knowledge requires no verification. When knowledge from the Super Conscious Wisdom comes into your awareness through a purified Conscience, you don't need an advanced degree—or any other special qualification—to know that the advice is indisputable. You intuitively know that it's true, and you *know* that you know. This is the knowledge that sets you free—if you can muster the will power to act on it.

Without regular use and purification, however, the Conscience may instead reflect only the limited perspectives of the Senses, the Ego and the Unconscious mind. This is a perfect example of the "squeaky wheel" theory. Sometimes the loud insistence of the Ego, Senses, memories, imagination, fear, anger and selfish desires can become the sole basis upon which the Conscience makes a decision. So, our task is to quiet the distracting noise in order to better hear the priceless signal of the Conscience. This is an essential step in coordinating all Four Functions of the Mind so that we can experience our highest good. I will offer some specific suggestions for how to experiment with this process in later chapters.

Before we move on, though, let's go back again to the hub of the wheel in our diagram. If you remember, the hub is your essential, eternal identity: *Sat-Chit-Ananda*. It is eternal. It is awareness. It is consciousness and wisdom. It is bliss, fullness and contentment. It is your Super Conscious Wisdom. Your Essential Nature. But just for a moment, consider that the same Essential Nature that is you, a human being, is also the same Essential Nature of all animals, plants and minerals. (Not to mention all other humans as well!) In fact, consciousness is all that really exists. It is both the cause and the substance of the material universe. Every transitory object that appears does so within that Awareness—including the human body and mind—with its thoughts, desires, emotions and concepts. The truth is, we really are all One. An acceptance of this Truth, in every decision we make, leads us to experience an unbounded compassion for all. It leads to Love, Fearlessness and Strength. More on that later!

For now, if we seek creative solutions for the many challenges that we face on any given day, our assignment is to purify our own Conscience and to parent the Senses, Ego, and Unconscious mind. As this process continues from relationship to relationship, all three of these functions of the mind will discover, through their own personal experience, that it is in their best interest to willingly serve the Super Conscious Wisdom reflected by the Conscience. If we are earnest and determined, we can train the mind to do this. It may not be easy at first, *but I assure you, from my own personal experience, that it is possible.* Your Conscience holds the key to unlocking your hidden potential for solving all of life's challenges.

Now let's take a closer look at how the *Buddhi,* your Conscience, decides whether any proposed action would lead to merely passing pleasure, or toward perennial joy.

CHAPTER 3

# Preya-Shreya-Buddhi-Ahimsa

*The voice of the conscience is so delicate*
*that it is easy to stifle it;*
*but it is also so clear that it is*
*impossible to mistake it.*

MADAME DE STAEL

Many of us are familiar with the world of Walt Disney and the insightful character of Jiminy Cricket. You might remember his cheerful advice to his truth-challenged student, Pinocchio, "Let your Conscience be your guide!"

In many respects, decision-making really is that simple. For thousands of years women and men have experimented with employing and respecting the Conscience as their personal, always-available, ever-reliable guide in choosing their best thoughts, words, and actions. Their method meant that the principle of *ahimsa* dictated kindness and diligence in every relationship—with themselves and with others. And what did they discover by regularly using their Conscience? They felt better physically, mentally, emotionally and spiritually. Old wounds healed, healthy relationships grew even stronger, and new, rewarding ones were born. They experienced the great gift of finding and serving a higher purpose in all of life.

But let's be honest, when we are out in the world living our lives, bumping up against all those gross and subtle objects (people, thoughts, desires and fears, for instance) it is often anything but easy to follow our Conscience. That doesn't make it any less worth the effort, and of course you already know this. Your very own Conscience has motivated you to read this book rather than watch TV, even if you could not have articulated that thought yet. And remember, through the process of purifying your Conscience (the *Buddhi*), you will become ever more aware of your Essential Nature. Some call it the Soul. We have called it your Super Conscious Wisdom. *Sat-Chit-Ananda*. Eternal consciousness, wisdom, fullness, and bliss. Whatever name you use, that inner light has always been there, glowing. It is Love, and that Love is what religions refer to as God, inside each of us.

# CONSCIENCE
## How You Receive Inner Wisdom

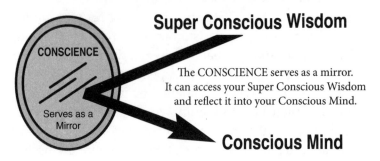

**Super Conscious Wisdom**

CONSCIENCE

Serves as a Mirror

The CONSCIENCE serves as a mirror. It can access your Super Conscious Wisdom and reflect it into your Conscious Mind.

**Conscious Mind**

Let's look at the important function that your Conscience, or *Buddhi*, serves relative to that inner light. The *Buddhi* is the instrument through which your conscious mind (the portion of the mind we are aware of) can access the intuitive library of knowledge from your Super Conscious Wisdom. When regularly exercised, the *Buddhi* becomes sharp and clear, like a brilliant mirror. But when it is ignored, it gets dusty and cloudy, and the other functions of the mind—that strong-willed Ego, those pleasure-seeking Senses, and all those Unconscious habits, memories, dreams, and fears—easily overpower it.

Purifying the *Buddhi* (your Conscience) is essential. You can cleanse and clarify the *Buddhi* through working on the experiments at the end of this book. And later, perhaps, you'll learn to practice seated meditation and various forms of "meditation-in-action" to help you act skillfully when you find yourself in an emotionally difficult situation. These practices will greatly enhance your ability to tap into ever higher levels of your Super Conscious Wisdom. And that, as Einstein advised us, is where the solutions to life's most difficult challenges will be found. As a bonus, joy resides there too—*Ananda*, that perfect contentment, fullness and bliss that is part of your Essential Nature. It is right there, waiting for you to discover it by sincerely engaging with these practices.

But please! Do not forget to be kind to yourself as you embark on this journey. Chances are pretty good that you won't go from zero to sixty overnight. Very few of us do. We must be patient and trust that the results will come in due time. They will. I assure you. And very often, if we are paying attention, we notice subtle changes in our energy right away, enough to help us find the motivation to keep experimenting. It is a beautiful process. For now, let us endeavor to understand more precisely what it means to "let your Conscience be your guide."

You learned in the last chapter that the Conscience is the only function of the mind that has the ability to see clearly and make a decision regarding any action that we may take. You also understand the mechanics behind the Law of Karma, which instruct that it is not possible for an action (and the resulting consequences) to occur without the occurrence, first, of a thought. Remember that you think 60,000-80,000 thoughts every day, and that most of them are the same ones you thought yesterday. Your thoughts are the most powerful natural resource available to you to attain your purpose in life. As William Jennings Bryan observed, "Destiny is not a matter of chance, it is a matter of choice." Therefore, in order to determine which thoughts to pay attention to, you must understand the nature and consequence of individual thoughts.

More than five thousand years ago, the wisdom of Yoga philosophy was revealed to ancient seers through meditation. It was recorded in scriptures that became known as the *Upanishads*. The Sanskrit word *Upanishad* literally means "to sit down near;" that is, to sit in front of a Guru to receive some important teaching.

In one of the principal *Upanishads*, the *Katha Upanishad*, the sages tell us that every thought falls into one of only two basic categories. That's right—there are only two kinds of thoughts! In the face of every circumstance you ever encounter—whether personal or professional, with family or strangers, in a fearful or loving situation—you are capable of thinking only two kinds of thoughts: the *preya* and the *shreya*.

*Preya* is defined as any thought that leads to short-term Ego or sense gratification, but that conflicts with our inner intuitive wisdom. Ah, *preya*! It's pleasant, attractive, familiar, comfortable and extremely easy to give our attention to. Our five Senses of sight, smell, taste, hearing, and touch are constantly investigating the objects of the material world in search of the pleasant. When our Senses identify something new and interesting, they immediately transmit the vital information back to our awareness, and we are flooded with thoughts that beckon us toward short-term gratification.

We are all very familiar with *preya*. In the realm of food choices, it's the candy bar. Related to daily exercise, it's the couch. Emotionally, the *preya* might be represented by worry, anger, fear, or selfishness—directed at yourself or others. *Preya* reflects a strong attachment; the ground upon which your personality currently stands. When you give your attention to the *preya*, you experience a spike of passing pleasure or satisfaction, but ultimately no long-term benefit. In fact, the passing pleasure of serving the *preya* is always followed by some form of contraction, pain or dis-ease. Fortunately, Yoga Science provides an alternative.

The second kind of thought that appears in our awareness is the *shreya*. The *shreya* is always in harmony with our inner wisdom, and its nature is expansive. Initially, the *shreya* may not be very pleasant, attractive, comfortable, or familiar to us. But the choice of *shreya* inevitably becomes deeply satisfying because it always leads toward lasting joy. In the food category, it's the carrots. Emotionally, it might appear as compassion or forgiveness.

If the *shreya* always leads to the highest and greatest good, and the *preya* eventually leads to some physical, mental, emotional or spiritual dis-ease, the choice for the Yoga Scientist is clear: every thought, word and action must be in service to the *shreya*. That is the black-and-white ideal, but in a world that appears in endless shades of gray, how, you ask, can you identify which thoughts are *preya* and which are *shreya*?

You will not be surprised to learn that your Super Conscious Wisdom always knows, and your purified Conscience has the power to reflect that wisdom and help you make the right decision. When the *Manas* presents us with choices that echo the calls of the Senses, Ego, and the Unconscious mind, the purified Conscience will unerringly define and endorse the *shreya*—the choice that will lead us for our highest and greatest good.

So if the Conscience is always directing us, and we already know what to do, why is it so difficult to hear the message? Can't we just turn up the volume? If only it were that easy. The voice of the Conscience is quiet, but it is also consistent and unmistakable. Thankfully, the science of sound engineering offers a key concept related to the interplay of signal and noise. To maximize the volume of a signal that cannot be enhanced, an engineer finds a way to lessen or eliminate the interfering noise. When the ambient noise level is lowered, the important signal becomes relatively more audible.

An historic example of this concept occurred during the Cold War in the 1950s, when the United States Information Agency broadcast news and rock 'n roll music throughout Eastern Europe. Although the signal was transmitted 24 hours a day, seven days a week, many people in Eastern European countries like Hungary, Czechoslovakia, Poland and East Germany rarely heard it. Why? Because the Soviet Union employed sophisticated electronics to jam the signal. They effectively found a way to turn up the noise and drown out the signal that the Americans were broadcasting.

Yoga Science recognizes a parallel in human life. The collective noisy opinions of the Senses, Ego and the memories and habits of the Unconscious mind are often so loud that they drown out the capacity of the Conscience to reflect wisdom from the center of consciousness. In order to hear the signal of your Super Conscious Wisdom and to heed its message, the Yoga Scientist must learn to turn down the noise of the Senses, the Ego and the Unconscious.

Learning to control and direct our one-pointed attention accomplishes this. That's why a daily meditation practice, ultimately, can prove to be so useful. There are many other strategies one can employ to turn down distracting noise, however. Experiments like the ones presented at the end of this book can be practiced before one learns to meditate. We might even think of them as "warm-up" exercises. They will help to establish your clear understanding of the Four Functions of the Mind and the essential role of the Conscience. Such an understanding leads to a life of joy, security, and meaning, a life filled with loving, fulfilling relationships.

Let's look at one last illustration to illuminate the importance of coordinating the Four Functions of the Mind in service to our Essential Identity. This one comes from the same scripture that gave us the two categories of thoughts—the *preya* (that which leads to passing pleasure) and the *shreya* (that which leads to everlasting joy).

The *Katha Upanishad* presents the story of a teenager named Nachiketa who sought enlightenment by asking life's most perplexing questions: Who am I? From where have I come? Why am I here? What is to be done? Where will I go?

Our body, the scripture says, is like a chariot drawn by five powerful horses, the five Senses. These horses gallop from birth toward death along the roads of desire, pursuing objects and relationships in hope of finding happiness and eliminating pain. The Conscience (*Buddhi*) is the charioteer, whose job it is to ensure that we're not pulled over a cliff by unrestrained horses. The reins held by the charioteer represent the mind with its many thoughts and emotions. And you, the Eternal Witness, the Divine Self, are the ever-present passenger—the true Master of the chariot.

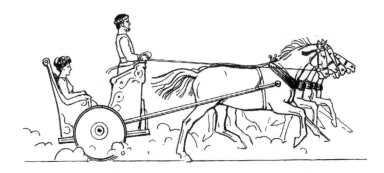

This poetic metaphor presents a number of practical implications. First and foremost, it's the role of the Conscience to keep you headed in the best direction. Its infallible wisdom skillfully controls the reins of the mind to steer the Senses along the roads of desire and move you toward your highest and greatest good. When all the major functions of the mind are coordinated to work in harmony, the real Self makes all the decisions. The Conscience, reflecting the will of the Supreme Intelligence, communicates this wisdom to the mind, and the Senses and body obey. But when the Senses are uncontrolled, they immediately take to the road of desire that promises immediate pleasure. In such circumstances, we clearly are not determining our destiny. We find ourselves, instead, enslaved to the whims of our horses.

With a bit of practice, a Yoga Scientist can always identify which function of the mind is presenting information into his or her awareness. For genuine health and happiness, these four faculties of your mind need to be coordinated and placed in service to the Higher Self, the hub of the wheel. The Senses, Ego and Unconscious mind must each do their job, but not more. Trusting that the purified Conscience alone can reflect the Super Conscious Wisdom of the Supreme Reality, you can lovingly parent the Four Functions of the Mind. Imagine all Four Functions of the

Mind as siblings vying for attention as they sit together with you, their parent, around the kitchen table to learn how to support the wisdom of the Conscience. No one is cast aside in this family engagement. It is simply a matter of learning to play well together. As this new collaboration becomes standard practice, we'll naturally serve the *shreya* and willingly surrender the *preya* in thought, word and deed—knowing the consequence will always be what you, the Ego, Senses and Unconscious mind really need.

Initially, this process might seem cumbersome, but soon you will create a global skill that enables you to make beneficial choices with a brilliance of confidence. This form of internal dialogue is very helpful. It teaches the mind, through personal experience, to take skillful actions that lead to the blessings of a joyful, creative, rewarding life.

To a great extent, the effectiveness of Yoga Science depends on your remembrance of your Essential Nature in every circumstance, and it is your Conscience that will help you remember. I have a body. I have a mind. I have thoughts, desires and emotions. I have an Ego and Unconscious mind. But the real "me" is not defined by these. Which takes us back to Nachiketa's first question: Who am I? The body, mind, Senses and Ego have manifested to serve our true identity, the Eternal Witness. Pure Consciousness. *Sat-Chit-Ananda.* When a human being knows and serves this Witness, the small, separate self becomes an instrument of the Supreme Intelligence. An instrument of God. When we do not follow the light of intuitive wisdom, however, we condemn ourselves to living in the darkness of ignorance, separateness, lack and pain.

So you see, these important teachings really can be boiled down to just four concepts: *preya, shreya, Buddhi,* and *ahimsa.* Remember them and you will find yourself on the same rewarding path as Nachiketa. Our young friend's spiritual inquiry was no mere intellectual or philosophical exercise. Rather, it was meant to challenge and inspire each of us to put an end to the suffering and alienation wrought by our doubts and fears. According to the scripture, this liberation is accomplished by experimenting with Yoga Science in order to experience the eternal, bliss-filled Supreme Reality for ourselves, in this lifetime. This realization, the sages tell us, is the only freedom worth attaining—the very purpose of our lives.

Now that you are familiar with the two different kinds of thoughts and the complex and brilliant nature of the mind that thinks them, let's tackle the business of how we actually go about training the mind. How do we get everybody to agree while sitting around the table? Managing our thoughts is a daily occurrence that none of us can escape—and why would we want to? Many of our thoughts are the expression of Divine Wisdom! We just need a few pointers for spotting and pulling out the weeds that inevitably appear in our human thought-gardens.

CHAPTER 4

# *The Power of Attention*

*If you bring forth what is within you,
what you bring forth will save you.*

*If you do not bring forth what is within you,
what you do not bring forth will destroy you.*

JESUS THE CHRIST
FROM THE GNOSTIC GOSPEL OF THOMAS

The first time you read the above statement, attributed to Jesus the Christ in the Gnostic Gospel of Thomas, written nearly 2,000 years ago, the words may seem puzzling. When you examine them in the light of the still older Science of Yoga, however, their profound and practical message becomes clear: our destiny depends on our ability to discover, manage and honor the tremendous power of our own minds. Access to our Super Conscious Wisdom can indeed assure that our lives will be purposeful and rewarding, but when we ignore or refuse that power, our resulting lack of love, courage, good judgment and creativity will inevitably diminish all our relationships—even contributing to the destruction of our beloved physical bodies.

As Yoga Scientists, we understand that all reality flows from the subtle to the gross. This Truth describes the mechanics underpinning the Law of Karma: thoughts (very subtle objects) lead to actions, and actions lead to consequences. This law of cause and effect is as real and unavoidable as the Law of Gravity.

We all make thousands of choices every day: what to eat, how much time to spend at work, at play, with family; how we choose the words we speak; how courteous we will be to others while driving or waiting in line at the grocery store. As you now understand, each of these choices begins with a thought. Yoga Science teaches us to recognize the nature of our thoughts (*preya* or *shreya*), and to understand our thought process. Through this aware- ness we learn that in any situation, we are best served by slowing down and creating some space between stimulus and response—rather than speaking the first words that come to mind, or bursting into action the moment a thought appears. In other words, by being more thought- ful about our thoughts, we become better able to make skillful and rewarding choices that lead to skillful and rewarding action in all circumstances.

These days, our culture does not encourage this kind of thoughtfulness. Rather, busy-ness is celebrated and instant gratification is the sought-after prize. Our minds are rarely calm and in the present moment, so many of our choices are not based on our own Inner Wisdom, but on the shortsighted or faulty perspectives of the Senses, Ego, and Unconscious mind. When we make choices based on this limited input, rather than on the Super Conscious Wisdom reflected by the Conscience/*Buddhi*, the con- sequences are more likely to bring pain to us, our families, communities, nation, and to the good Earth, our Mother.

How, then, do we become loving stewards of our own

minds? How do we learn to evaluate our thoughts in order to bring about harmony and peace, rather than suffering, in all our relationships,? This is our highest calling.

I have found it useful to consider individual thoughts as tiny embryos, and our attention as an incubator employed in the process of creation. When you give attention to a thought, that subtle embryo is incubated. When sufficient attention has been given, a concrete form of the thought-object is born into the material world. The more you think a thought, the more likely you are to speak about that thought. With sustained attention to the same thought, you're likely to undertake some physical action in the material world that can successively create ever more complex relationships—all in service to that original embryo called a thought. Both the words and the actions are concrete manifestations of that subtle thought-embryo you nurtured with your attention.

Let's assume that a specific thought comes into your awareness. No one else is aware of this particular thought, just you. Others, of course, have their own thoughts that you are not aware of. You have received this specific thought now, in the present moment. At this point in space and time you are present in a unique constellation of relationships throughout the universe, and your mind-body-sense complex is the only one perfectly qualified to take some action in response to this subtle thought-object appearing in your awareness. So it has come to you. Your job is to decide what to do with that thought.

Every thought is only a suggestion. It is not an imperial command. If, in the present moment, your Conscience advises you that the thought, desire or emotion in your awareness is a *shreya*, give it your complete attention. Remember, a *shreya* is one of the two kinds of thoughts we are capable of having; the *shreya* always leads us for our highest and greatest good. This message from the Conscience means that you have been chosen, from among the billions of people in the world, to incubate this thought-embryo that the Supreme Intelligence (through your own Super Conscious Wisdom) is bringing forth from the subtle world. Your capacity to focus attention on that thought, in the present moment—now—is the Divine mechanism for transforming the subtle thought-object into manifest form. This progression from the subtle thought to the more concrete forms of speech, action and consequence is the process of creation. By aligning every thought, word and action with the infinite wisdom of the Conscience, you become an instrument of the Supreme Reality in the process of creation.

What an awesome honor and responsibility! Perhaps you have had the sense that some greater force is working through you when you are fully engrossed in a particularly meaningful task or relationship. It might be connected to your professional life, or it might happen when you are bathing your child, or caring for your elderly parent. It may have lasted for only a moment, but you can learn how to sustain this sense of purpose and meaning in your daily experience.

In Hindu literature, Krishna is the personification of the longing that spiritual seekers feel in their own hearts, the yearning that draws them into a deeper relationship with the Divine. It is no different from a Christian's relationship with the Christ that lives within. Krishna—strong, beautiful and charismatic—is often depicted playing a hollow reed flute. The seeker who can purify the body, mind and Senses by renouncing attachments to fear, anger and self-willed desire becomes the instrument through which the Divine melody is played. When we listen to the Conscience and give our attention to the thought-object that is the *shreya*, we are joining that beautiful symphony.

St. Francis taught, "It is in dying (to the separate sense of self), that we are born to eternal life." Many writers have defined Yoga Science and meditation as the "art of dying"—learning how to die to our attachments before we have to die physically. As we learn to unencumber ourselves of our limitations, we can "become One with the Father (the Supreme Intelligence) who is in heaven" and experience *turiya*—the fourth state of consciousness beyond waking, dreaming and deep sleep. This is the state of tranquility and equanimity that sages of various traditions have called *moksha* (liberation), Christ-consciousness, nirvana or the land of milk and honey.

But for now let's get back to the familiar, ordinary world we must navigate daily.

Of the tens of thousands of thoughts that you think every day, not all of them will lead you beyond pain and bondage, to ultimate freedom. Often, when you become aware of a thought, desire, or emotion, the quiet voice of the Conscience suggests to you that it is a *preya*, not a *shreya*. The *preya*, you remember, is the category of thought that leads first to passing pleasure, but eventually to some form of pain—not perennial joy. And as you've learned, the Conscience always knows the difference.

Let's look at an example. You might spend several days rehashing an argument you had with your child/parent/teacher/friend/boss, going over it again and again in your mind, always reaching the same conclusion: you were completely misunderstood. You recognize that compulsively replaying this emotionally-charged memory is not leading to resolution, but you can't seem to stop—even though your Conscience has advised that it's a *preya*. You now have three clear choices of what to do with your attention: You can continue to give your attention to the attractively familiar *preya*. But if you do, the *preya* will eventually manifest as some form of physical, mental or emotional dis-ease or pain.

You may repress the *preya*. However, repressed energy will eventually manifest as a destructive, painful neurosis.

The only desirable choice for a Yoga Scientist is to surrender the *preya*.

What do I mean by surrender the *preya*? Let's go back for a moment and consider that every tiny thought-embryo comes to us for some distinct, positive purpose—regardless of whether it is a *shreya* or *preya*. If the Conscience says it's a *shreya*, you know to serve it through your speech and action, and you'll be led for your highest and greatest good. But if the Conscience says it's a *preya*, Yoga Science teaches us to surrender it back to your personal concept of the Supreme Intelligence.

That thought, like all thoughts, is simply energy, and while energy cannot be created nor destroyed, it can be transformed into strategic reserves of healing energy, will power and creativity that will enable you to fulfill the purpose of your life. That's right—when you surrender the *preya*, you will experience an increase in energy, will power and creativity. These reserves, stored in a potential state, can be accessed at another time to perform any demanding responsibility the Conscience suggests. This transformational process is not fiction. It is a practical, scientific, reproducible methodology you can use to solve even the most difficult challenges you face.

So when the Conscience advises you that a thought is a *preya*, willingly and lovingly surrender it. Here is a prayer that you might find useful:

*"O Inner Dweller, I hear the Conscience telling me that this thought is a preya. I earnestly and humbly offer this thought and its emotional turmoil back to you, the Origin of all. Please accept this offering as the loving gift of a dedicated heart.*

*Consume it in the fire of your Light, purify my instrument that I might do Thy will, and lead me for my highest, greatest good."*

With practice, you will quickly become more skillful at recognizing the voice and wisdom of the Conscience when it advises that a thought is a *preya*. I advise you to start small, with the obvious *preyas*, like the cup of caffeinated coffee right before bedtime. Can you think of other examples? Learning to sacrifice the *preya* demands the same process required to cultivate any new skill—practice, practice, practice. *The challenge is to develop sufficient will power until a new habit is formed.* The more you do it, the more it reinforces your ability and your desire to do it. When you are successful with the easy choices, you'll automatically be building your will power for the more difficult ones. Being mindful of this process will also keep you centered in your Essential Nature, a state of mind that improves your performance of any task you undertake.

On the other hand, if you ignore (or forget) your Divine Nature at the moment a thought, desire or emotion appears in your awareness, you're more likely to disregard or overlook the wise and good counsel of the Conscience and be swayed by the siren call of the Senses, Ego and Unconscious mind. You may even be fooled temporarily into believing that you're choosing the *preya* through your own free will, but remember that actions chosen on the basis of fear, anger and self-willed desire will always result in dis-ease.

A purified Conscience will always encourage you to serve the *shreya*. Disregarding the Conscience, however, and serving the *preya* in thought, word or deed amounts to subtle violence against the unique thought-embryo (*shreya*) that the Supreme Reality has suggested you bring forth into the material world.

To help us grasp the harm in this potential action, let's

consider the idea of abortion. Remember, we are not talking about a human embryo, and I am aware of the emotionally charged nature of the word abortion. But it is a helpful analogy for a critical concept, so I ask that you acknowledge any emotions that may have surfaced, surrender them, and then re-center yourself in your Essential Nature. Bring your attention back to the present moment, free from any unhelpful preconceptions.

In a sense, each of us (including me) is regularly guilty of inflicting violence, of not practicing *ahimsa*. Many times a day we betray our Conscience and abort potential manifestations of *shreya*. When we ignore the counsel of the Conscience and withhold our attention from the tiny thought-embryo that is the *shreya*, that thought-embryo dies. Any positive words, actions or consequences that may have resulted from it die along with it. Our karmas change. The world changes. And not for the better.

The physical, mental and emotional pain rampant in our society, and our futile reliance on remedies such as pharmacology, consumerism, the penal system, and the military to ameliorate the dis-ease, can be viewed yogically as direct consequences of the violence we inflict individually and collectively on the Conscience and the many *shreyas* we chose not to serve. When the principle of *ahimsa* is disregarded, the resulting action inevitably has an injurious effect.

Now, without judgment, imagine that a woman becomes pregnant and that the fetus is aborted sometime during the gestation period. This does not mean that the woman cannot give birth to a child at some future time. In all likelihood she will be able to have another child. However, she will never give birth to the child she lost.

Similar rules apply to our thoughts. If, in the present moment, we receive a thought that the Conscience defines as *shreya*, the Supreme Intelligence is asking us to give this particular thought our full attention in order to facilitate the birth of its more concrete form. But we have free will. We can choose not to participate further in developing the form of this subtle embryo. We can ignore or forget it. We can let it die.

We can and will receive another thought, or perhaps even the very same thought, in the future. At that point in space and time, however, a new constellation of relationships will exist—one entirely different from that which existed at the time of the first thought. It is simply impossible to go back in time and resurrect a *shreya* that has been lost. That is why living in the present moment and staying open to the *shreya* is essential to our health and well-being. If our conscious attention is not focused in the now, we will miss the message of the Conscience, continue to serve the *preya*, and thus remain enslaved in a whirlpool of painful consequences.

This is not to suggest, in any way, that Yoga Scientists must deny themselves the enjoyments of the world. Quite the contrary! Through the practice of Yoga Science (including the simple experiments with the Conscience offered in Chapters 6 and 7,) you will become even more free and prepared to experience the world joyously and rewardingly.

We have a body and Senses, and life is to be enjoyed, but it is only by staying true to our Super Conscious Wisdom, that precious treasure buried within each of us, that the world can be fully appreciated. Only with an exercised and purified Conscience can the human being become truly happy, healthy, creative, productive, artistic, loving and nurtured to the fullest extent. Therefore, if what you had hoped and planned for is fulfilled, be grateful. If what you had hoped and planned for is *not* fulfilled, be equally grateful, as long as you have served the *shreya* and sacrificed the *preya*. Through your own experience, and despite the protests of the Ego, Senses and Unconscious Mind, you will come to know that you are indeed being led for your highest and greatest good.

## How to Purify the Conscience/*Buddhi* and Optimize Your Wisdom

Building your capacity to recognize and listen to your Conscience, which functions as a mirror, is essential to your ongoing ability to serve the *shreya* and sacrifice the *preya*. While the Conscience has no inherent wisdom of its own, it does have the ability to access your Super Conscious Wisdom and reflect it into the everyday operation of your conscious mind. However, unless a mirror is cleaned regularly, dust accumulates on its surface and obscures the mirror's reflective quality. Similarly, when you don't establish and maintain the habit of using your Conscience regularly, its ability to reflect the Truth from your Essential Nature is diminished.

In such cases, the Conscience still retains the power to discern, determine, judge and decide, but without access to your intuitive, inner wisdom, only the relatively loud and insistent voices of the Ego, Senses and Unconscious Mind can be heard and considered. As a result, the Conscience will still make the final decision about what to do and what not to do, but its decision will be made on the basis of limited and possibly faulty input.

However, and here is the good news, each time you heed your Conscience and sacrifice the *preya*, not only are you increasing your reserves of energy, will power and creativity, you're also cleaning the mirror that will guide you in every relationship and circumstance.

By offering your mind, action and speech in service to your Inner Wisdom, as reflected by your Conscience, you are no longer the author of a particular action, and therefore have no claim to its outcome. This act of renunciation is not a "quid pro quo"—you do not make this offering expecting a specific result. Remember, the word sacrifice comes from the Latin *sacrificium*, meaning to make sacred. Your willing sacrifice of the *preya* is an act of trustful surrender. Regardless of the consequence, earnest seekers always know they are being led for their highest and greatest good. For the Yoga Scientist, this option is the only acceptable choice.

You've probably seen some version of the old shell game. In this carnival trick you're asked to follow the pea under one of three moving walnut shells. A skillful operator can move the pea in the blink of an eye from one shell to another, and unless you're present in the moment and totally focused, you're likely to make the wrong choice. Of course, in real life situations our errors are not the fault of a deceitful operator, but rather the result of our own inattention. Unless you are present in the *now*, know your true Self, and can identify which function of the mind is presenting information, you may miss the Divine counsel of the Conscience.

Please remember this important point: what is clearly the *shreya* on one occasion might become the *preya* on the next. And what is *preya* in one particular circumstance may well become the *shreya* in another. Consider your desire for a slice of apple pie, for example. Let's say that apple pie represents one of your strongest food desires. If you've enjoyed a special dinner at a friend's home and you're offered a slice of homemade apple pie for dessert, the Conscience might appropriately suggest that it is the *shreya*. After all, life is to be enjoyed, and this is your favorite! Besides, if your host has lovingly prepared apple pie especially for you, it might not be kind to refuse the thoughtful gesture. However, if you're offered a second piece of apple pie ten minutes later, the Conscience will probably advise that this second slice is clearly a *preya*.

Are there any guidelines for determining whether a particular thought is a *shreya* or *preya*? Remember that your Super Conscious Wisdom already has the answer. Every time. Still, you might find the following brief outline helpful as you undertake the process of tapping into that wisdom when you are faced with a choice that is more difficult than whether or not to have the second slice of pie:

**1. Be focused in the moment.**

**2. Center yourself** in the fullness of your Essential Nature (*Sat-Chit-Ananda*).

**3. Recognize which function of the mind** (your Senses, Ego, or Unconscious mind) is authoring a particular thought.

**4. Listen to the voice of your Conscience/*Buddhi*.** As you concentrate on the Conscience with one-pointed attention, the noise of the Senses, Ego and Unconscious mind will become relatively quiet.

**5. Face the challenge.** Upon hearing the Divine wisdom reflected by the Conscience, surrender attachment to the *preya*, sacrifice it, and, with all the will power you can summon, align every thought, word and action with the wise and good counsel of the Conscience. Serve the *shreya* with all your heart.

**6. Repeat, repeat, repeat with every choice!**

It takes strength, courage and will power to harmonize mind, action and speech with the Conscience. You may have to go against the tide of our culture and the habits of a lifetime. While the Conscience is always defining the *shreya*, the Senses, Ego and Unconscious mind may very well be attempting to jam that signal, just like the Soviets did back in the Cold War. Meanwhile, the advertising industry sometimes generates bogus promises that sing the praises of the *preya*, reinforcing the notion that you are a separate entity in search of other separate entities that can make you happy and eliminate your pain.

Unless we're deliberately serving the wisdom reflected by a purified Conscience, we are all susceptible to the pitch. When conflict exists in the mind, it can be difficult to maintain the focused attention needed to evaluate each suggestion in the moment. But if we fail to make the effort, our habits (those channels in the "wet sand" of the Unconscious mind) determine our actions, and we unconsciously deny ourselves the happy, healthy, joyful life we so deeply desire. Remember this Truth: each one of us, including you, has the power to access that beautiful life. Doesn't that make it worth the effort?

CHAPTER 5

# The Bridge of Yoga:
# Outer Actions and Inner Wisdom

*Inner wisdom is more important than wealth.*
*The more you spend, the more you gain.*

OPRAH WINFREY

The realization of a happy, healthy and joyful life begins with the recognition that you are a citizen of two worlds. Clearly, you are a citizen of the ever-changing material world of animal, vegetable and mineral matter. In this familiar environment, the body is your vehicle for action and your mind is your most powerful instrument for evaluating circumstances and motivating your body into action. By now you know that for every action your mind-body-sense complex takes, a consequence results.

You also understand that you are a citizen of the distinctly non-material, yet profoundly real world of consciousness. Remember the answer to that all important question, "Who Am I?" At the core of your being you are *Sat-Chit-Ananda*: an eternal being, pure consciousness, wisdom, and bliss. This is your Essential Nature, your true unchanging Self. Within this transcendent world exists the intuitive library of higher knowledge that unerringly identifies which of your possible actions will lead you to realize health, happiness and freedom from fear, and which will lead to physical, mental, emotional and spiritual disease. Your *Conscience* is the key to accessing that knowledge.

The challenge is to remember your higher Self when you are at the grocery store, in a meeting at work, or sitting home alone on a Friday night. It is a continual process of remembering and forgetting, remembering and forgetting, then remembering again. One could say that our goal is to remember our higher Self on a more regular basis, when we are out in the material world (including our own home) making choices, engaging in communication, and performing actions. *When, as a citizen of the world, your outer actions reflect the perfection of your inner, subtle wisdom, you will be led for your highest and greatest good.* This choice—to base your outer action on your own inner wisdom—is the essence of all forms of yoga. We call this process the *Bridge of Yoga*. Yoga means union, and the Science of Yoga provides a reliable blueprint for building a trustworthy, ever-accessible bridge to your own inner wisdom.

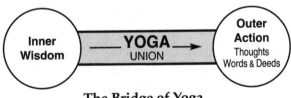

### The Bridge of Yoga

Yoga means union. It represents a bridge between your Inner Wisdom and your outer actions. When your thoughts, words and deeds are based on the Inner Wisdom accessed by the Conscience, you are always led for your highest and greatest good. There is no cause for worry.

The *Bridge of Yoga* is a very practical tool that can be employed easily in every circumstance and relationship.

It is simply another way of understanding or visualizing what happens when we let our Conscience be our guide. The *Bridge of Yoga* is both a metaphor and a scientific template that has helped many people stay centered in their Essential Nature. By using it regularly, you can learn to deal confidently and skillfully with common, everyday situations. Take worrying for example.

Worry is neither genuine concern nor creative problem solving. Worry is the reptilian brain's insistence that some unexamined fear will lead to loss. Compulsive worrying is the misuse of our sacred energy. Yet to one extent or another, we all worry. If the truth were known, most of us squander a tremendous amount of creative energy attending to notions of what the future might or might not hold. Just as Gulliver was hopelessly bound by the Lilliputians' slender threads, many of us are held captive by habitual thoughts generated from our own fertile imaginations.

How alluring that unending train of hypothetical "what if" situations can be! "What if this should happen? What if that should happen? And what if neither happens?" So much of life is spent imagining things that never were and never will be. As Mark Twain put it, "I am an old man and have had many troubles, most of which never happened." Far too often, our concerns even prevent us from getting a good night's sleep. And the more attention we give our worries, the worse we feel—physically, mentally, emotionally and spiritually. This need not be the case.

Why? Because if you are a person who worries a great deal, or is often angered by situations and relationships, or besieged by desires for physical pleasure or material possessions, it means that you are a very wealthy individual. Your fears, anger and self-centered desires represent a powerful natural resource. Their latent power can bring you the health, happiness, creativity, productivity, fearlessness, and loving, nurturing relationships you seek—if you are willing to make use of your attention as an internal mechanism for transformation.

Imagine for a moment that you've discovered a vast deposit of gold ore in your backyard. Without employing a mining operation and processing plant, you'd never benefit from your potential wealth. Similarly, without a philosophy of life that can turn your *preyas* into usable energy, will power and creativity, you will never realize your greatest potential. With your newfound understanding of the Four Functions of the Mind, and your dedication to learning how to coordinate the Senses, Ego, and Unconscious mind to listen to the wisdom of the Conscience, you can transform that energy. It takes practice, but I am absolutely confident that you can do it.

This is a critical first understanding. But awareness is not enough. You need a plan of action. *The Bridge of Yoga* can help. When you have done all that you can do in a situation, but still find yourself plagued by worries, use this checklist to transform the power of those worrisome thoughts into reserves of energy, willpower and creativity. By surrendering the *preya*, you are building strength and resilience. Remember, perennial happiness is never realized by simply dismissing your concerns for the future, nor by repressing them. Rather, when you become a Yoga Scientist, you can face thoughts that tempt you to worry, as they arise, by experimenting with this gentle and loving time-tested procedure.

### First-Aid Kit for Worries — Using the Bridge of Yoga

1. Before you address your anxiety, pause and ask yourself the question, "Who am I?" Through this form of quiet contemplation, your attention becomes centered in

the peace and fullness of the Eternal Witness, your Perfect wisdom. This first step is the key to basing your outer actions on your inner wisdom. In time, it will become second nature to you.

2. To calm the mind, attend to the inhalation and exhalation of your breath at the bridge between the nostrils (where the nostrils meet the upper lip) for 60 seconds.

3. As you remain centered in the equanimity of the Eternal Witness, practice detachment and dispassionately welcome, witness and honor your concerns—allowing yourself to be present with these thoughts, desires and emotions without being controlled by them.

4. Listening to the inner wisdom of your Conscience, willingly surrender the worrisome thought (the *preya*) back to its Origin—the Origin of every person, every thing, and every thought (the Supreme Intelligence).

5. Try to recognize an opportunity (it's probably in front of you right now) to engage in some selfless service. It might be as simple as washing the dishes, or you could call or visit an elderly friend or relative. Selfless action will transform the energy of worry into the energy of love, fearlessness and strength.

6. Later, when you establish a seated meditation practice, you can strengthen the *Bridge of Yoga* by lovingly directing your attention to your mantra (the name of the Supreme Reality that you are most comfortable with). We'll talk more about this in the next book, or you can read about it in my book, *The Heart and Science of Yoga.*®

7. If it's possible, go for a brisk 15-20 minute walk, gently swinging your arms and focusing attention on your natural breath as you inhale and exhale.

8. Repeat steps one through seven as needed whenever you recognize that you are being plagued by worry.

Throughout history, the profound insights of Yoga Science and philosophy (such as this "First-Aid Kit for Worries") have been taught and re-experienced within the culture and idioms of changing times, so that their healing and nurturing effects can be embraced anew by each successive generation. Whenever their inner wisdom has been realized and relied upon, individuals have experienced the greatest freedom of all: the freedom from worry and fear. When you learn to embrace this freedom through a daily practice of Yoga Science, your life will become a great and meaningful adventure. On that journey, you naturally blossom to your fullest potential.

Because this ageless Truth is intrinsically universal and democratic, countless people have realized the freedom of enlightenment without ever hearing the word "Yoga" or knowing anything about Eastern philosophy. Yet, the science and philosophy of Yoga have always provided quiet, reliable encouragement and concrete guidance to seekers in every culture, tradition and religion.

If, even now, all the talk about basing your outer actions on your inner wisdom still sounds a little too pie-in-the-sky for you, it only means that you have a scientifically oriented mind that needs to verify any new hypothesis. Actually, there's a term for that kind of person. It's "Yoga Scientist." This book is written for you. My hope is that your curiosity has been tapped and that you will choose to spend some time playing with the experiments in the next chapter. I have never asked you to take my word for anything I've presented. Most of us need to experience something personally, often many times over, before we make the decision to internalize it and make any lasting changes to how we live our lives. I am this kind of a person myself, which is why I started experimenting all those decades ago when I was first introduced to Yoga Science. I was intrigued and inspired enough by the results to continue to experiment, and I believe you will be too.

Before you begin the experiments in the next two chapters, let's take a moment to review what we've covered. I recognize that these concepts, while ancient, may be completely new to you. And the Sanskrit terms might sound strange to your ears. However, I also know that you have stuck with it so far because it makes sense to you. It resonates somewhere deep within. As you have read the words on these pages, you understood exactly what was being conveyed. I know this because your Super Conscious Wisdom has been there all along, just waiting for you to find it. It is the work of my life to guide people to discover their higher Self, and I am pleased for you that you have chosen to direct your attention to the teachings that have been presented thus far.

## Summing It All Up—A Review

Yoga Science teaches us that in every relationship you can easily access your own inner wisdom to substantiate, or refute, any form of hearsay that you might be receiving from your Senses, your Ego, or your Unconscious mind. That's right—24 hours a day, 7 days a week, and 365 days of the year your Conscience is continuously broadcasting unerring wisdom from the Superconscious Mind—like a radio signal—into your conscious mind. The *Buddhi* is the Conscience, or in the language of early Christianity, it's the Holy Spirit. The Conscience is analogous to a mirror because, when it is used regularly to decide what's to be done and what's not to be done, it faithfully reflects the wisdom and will of the Supreme Reality (a.k.a. God).

The Conscience allows the conscious mind access to insights from the intuitive library of knowledge within— your Super Conscious Wisdom. When such knowledge enters the conscious mind, no verification of its truthfulness is necessary. When your Conscience speaks, you know what it says is true. The only question that remains is, do you have the will power to align every thought, word and action with the wise and good counsel of the Conscience?

The Superconscious Mind is not a figment of one's imagination. It is the same aspect of the mind from which Albert Einstein saw mathematical equations and Paul McCartney hears beautiful melodies. When you earnestly serve the quiet promptings of the Conscience, instead of exclusively serving the limited and habitual perspectives of the Senses, Ego and Unconscious mind, the Conscience, operating like a mirror, can reflect an appropriate aspect of Divine Wisdom into your conscious mind. By regularly listening to the Conscience and employing its suggestions in thought, word and deed, you will directly and positively enhance every relationship.

The word conscience comes from the Latin, and it means "with wisdom or knowledge." As a Yoga Scientist, you are simply asked to make all your decisions consciously—based on the science of Yoga and on the reliable advice of the Conscience.

The Conscience/*Buddhi* enables us to free ourselves from the pains, miseries and bondages created by our learned habits of fear, anger and greed. Yoga Scientists of long ago explain that each of us has been born to learn how to regularly use the infallible discrimination of the Conscience so that we might transcend the animal habits of our mind—through our capacities, now, as human beings—to unite with the Supreme Consciousness at the core of our being. And in any language, that translates into our ability to experience a happy, healthy, joyful life.

But here's the challenge. If we continue to accept the

overblown promises from the culture, Senses, habits or Ego—without exercising our best judgment as reflected by the Conscience—we will not always receive what was promised. And, if we continue disregarding our Super Conscious Wisdom, we will inevitably continue to experience forms of physical, mental, emotional or spiritual disease. The only way to know for certain if a particular thought will lead us for our highest and greatest good is to follow the wisdom of the mind's Conscience. When we employ the *Bridge of Yoga* and align every thought, word and physical action with our inner wisdom, our lives will become increasingly healthy, happy, creative, productive and free of the dis-ease of stress, anxiety and pain.

That is my prayer for you, that you come to know, through your own process of experimentation with the tools of Yoga Science, that you have the power to manifest your deepest driving desires. The world needs each one of us to bring our best Self forward. When we teach our minds to serve the *shreya* and sacrifice the *preya*, we become equipped to resolve not only our everyday challenges, but also the challenges that may have previously seemed unresolvable. And the truth is, every time we solve a small challenge creatively at home, it prepares us to solve those larger challenges out in the world. Even the biggest ones.

## A Higher Purpose

In today's culture, we are urged to move at excessive speed and react instantaneously, without taking time to examine our thoughts and evaluate what's best to be done and what's best *not* to be done. But the reassuring message from the ancient sacred text, the *Bhagavad Gita*, is clear and prophetic: "Whenever there is a decline of Truth and a rise of untruthfulness, the Supreme Intelligence appears in the human organism to protect and reestablish *dharma*—the Truth that will uphold and maintain the individual and collective social order and make it possible for humanity to flourish."

This Divine appearance is not a fantasy superhero that comes to earth with abilities far beyond those of mere mortals. Nor is it a force that reflects shallow, but popular, misunderstandings of scriptures and mythologies. Rather, because all the problems and pain caused by non-truth begin in the human mind, these problems can be solved only by purifying the human mind. The entire process of reestablishing the *dharma* begins when each of us starts understanding and coordinating The Four Functions of our own mind.

You have already begun to play your part. Thank you. As you continue to work to change your own consciousness, you will find that you begin to feel a connection to others, even those you do not know, that you may not have felt in the past. This connection naturally leads one to consider the purpose of one's life in a new light.

Some might say that the purpose of life is to know God. But that is not true. Those who claim that knowing God is the purpose of life have usually heard someone else make that assertion, and have accepted it as their own belief.

The sages of all traditions claim that the true purpose of life is to be free of the pains, miseries and bondages of human existence. "If you think you know God and have a relationship with the Divine," Swami Rama of the Himalayas taught, "but are still ravaged by pain, miseries, and bondages, of what use is that God? If, however, you are free from the sorrow of human existence, the sages would conclude that you have already found God."

The great value of this human life is that it provides both the capacity and the means to end our suffering. We now have a human body, mind, Senses and discriminative faculty—all the requisites for making the transition from the animal to the Divine. The sages promise that we can be free in this very lifetime. Further, they urge us not to postpone the endeavor. Enlightenment, they say, is our birthright—a state free from pains, miseries and bondages. It is not something to be acquired or something new. It is already within us. Each of us, therefore, can realize this state by transforming our habits and purifying our personalities. We have been granted this rare opportunity by Providence to make ourselves fit to receive our full inheritance. This is our challenge as human beings.

In order to be free from all limitations and to fulfill the purpose of your life, you must be your true Self and rely on the wisdom within to guide your actions in the world. If, however, you remain ignorant of the Supreme Intelligence within, your thoughts, words, and actions will remain enslaved to the power of the fear, anger and self-willed desires stored in the Unconscious mind, and you will continue to feel pain and discontent. The choice is yours.

### Contemplate the Question "Who am I?"

Every desire that motivated you to read this book and investigate Yoga Science can be fulfilled if you earnestly contemplate the question "Who am I?" This inquiry, called *vichara* in ancient yogic texts, has been esteemed for thousands of years as a reliable method of knowing the true Self. If you are sincere and persistent in posing this question to yourself, the answer will come. And, as the truth of that answer motivates you to steward the energy of your innumerable desires, large and small, you will begin to experience freedom from your fear, anger, anxiety and dis-ease.

This process occurs differently for each human being.

Guided by the philosophy of Yoga Science, you will begin to follow your own distinct path to Self-realization and freedom. Each of us has been born with a unique mind-body-sense complex, and through this vehicle each of us experiences a different reality. Yet, from that transitory individuality, each human being has the capacity to know union with the Divine.

Absolute peace and contentment is the fruit of earnestly seeking the answer to the profound question "Who am I?" The contemplation of this question begins with the systematic, step-by-step procedure to focus your mind. With this focus, you can transcend the indiscriminate call of the Senses and the Ego's fascination with the past or future. Then, as your mind becomes ever more focused, you will enter a timeless state as you become present to the joyful and creative possibilities of your own true nature.

Begin this practice by repeatedly asking yourself the question: Who am I? During the contemplation, remember this:

*I have a body. I am aware of the body, but I am not the body.*
*I have a mind. I am aware of the mind, but I am not the mind.*
*I have thoughts. I am aware of thoughts, but I am not thoughts.*
*I have desires. I am aware of desires, but I am not desires.*
*I have emotions. I am aware of emotions, but I am not emotions.*

*Who, then, is aware of the body?*
*Who is aware of the mind?*
*Who is aware of the thoughts, desires and emotions?*
*Who is the thinker of every thought?*
*Who is the experiencer of every experience?*
*Who am I?*

Beginning today, and for the rest of your life, contemplate the question "Who am I?" If you are earnest in your effort—allowing consciousness to observe conscious-ness—the answer will appear, because the question and the answer are two sides of the same coin.

Whenever there is consternation in your mind, you are reacting from the limited perspective of the personality. It's a clear indication that the Ego—not the real You—has its hands on the wheel of the bus. When thoughts, desires, emotions and concepts arise in your awareness, do not automatically pursue them with your attention, but rather, inquire: "To whom did this thought arise?" It doesn't matter how many thoughts arise. As each thought arises, inquire with diligence: "To whom has this thought arisen?" The answer that will emerge is: "To me." If you earnestly inquire "Who am I?" at this point, the mind will go deeper to consider its Source, and the thought that arose will become less seductive. Seeking the answer to the question "Who am I?" will eventually give rise to the realization that within you dwells an Eternal Witness which *is* the Supreme Reality.

This dialogue requires attentive introspection. Be sensitive and patient as you consider your feelings and thoughts. Be gentle with yourself, as you would with any good friend. Practice *ahimsa*. Don't condemn yourself or be judgmental, and you will begin to trust your inner Self and realize that a constantly faithful companion and guide resides within.

As the profound Truth begins to unfold, you will find that everything you need in order to fulfill your life's purpose will spontaneously appear, and the objects and relationships that do not serve your highest good will begin to fall away. This means that your life will gradually become uncluttered, unstressed, vibrant, productive and creative. As old habits drop away, you will find yourself increasingly free to explore new possibilities.

CHAPTER 6

# Experimenting with Your Conscience

*The deeper your search in the mine of truth,
the richer the discovery of the gems buried there.*

MAHATMA GANDHI

*People who say it cannot be done
should not interrupt those who are doing it.*

GEORGE BERNARD SHAW

Early in the 1920s Mahatma Gandhi was working to promote civil rights in South Africa, and one evening he was traveling alone by train. He was a highly educated young attorney, well-dressed and seated in first-class accommodations. A British conductor approached him and announced that because of his dark skin he would have to move to the rear coach. Gandhi insisted that he had appropriate first-class passage, displayed his ticket and refused to submit to the racist indignity. Despite his protestations, however, young Gandhi was summarily thrown off the train.

That night in a cold, dark, abandoned railroad station, Gandhi was battered by a relentless storm of rage. He endured wave after wave of fury as he strode up and down the platform, fuming. Mighty, righteous anger roared in his awareness throughout the night, raising the level of his wrath to volcanic proportions.

Now, Gandhi could have reacted in a destructive manner. He could have chosen to serve the *preya*. He could have picked up a club or found a gun. He could have injured or even killed someone. Instead, recalling the Truth of Yoga Science, Gandhi had a profound realization that night: Anger is power!

At that time in history India was still under the colonial rule of the British Empire, and the Indian people were angry about it. In the midst of his own rage, Gandhi suddenly recognized the tremendous power that existed in the collective anger of his people—enough power, if it were creatively transformed and focused, to cast off the shackles of the world's greatest military force. In one great flash of insight, Gandhi knew that his vision for Indian independence could be realized by transforming huge reserves of angry, mental energy—through the disciplined practice of *ahimsa*, non-violence. He had found his purpose.

Gandhi's ability to recognize anger as a source of power can inspire and instruct us to utilize this potent mechanism for resolving our own persistent challenges. And it is not just anger that can be transformed; worry and anxiety are also reliable sources of potential creative energy. By coupling a strong *shreya* desire with your one-pointed attention, you too can facilitate wonders in your own life. The key is turning abstract theory into practice. The experiments in this chapter will get you started, and as you might guess, it all begins with your Conscience.

One of the most meaningful ways you can experience the benefits of your Super Conscious Wisdom is to experiment by committing to use your own Conscience when deciding which thoughts to think, words to speak and actions to take. Remember, your Conscience knows that not everything you "like" is good for you, and that everything you "dislike" isn't always bad for you. If you begin by experimenting with small, relatively easy decisions, almost immediately you will feel more positive about yourself, more self-confident, self-reliant, and grateful for the love and kindness you are offering to yourself and to the world. Pay close attention to if and how your mental and emotional attitudes change when you become quiet and focused enough to hear the voice of the Conscience. Then, in that state of equanimity, heed your own intuitive wisdom. Throughout your experimentation practice, keep a journal of your observations, reflections and the consequences that develop from your choices. You will find this very helpful.

## Experiment 1
## Food Empowers the Mind and Body

Desire is the fuel for action, and actions have consequences. Your desire for food is what motivates you to eat, and eating assures the continuation of your life. But not every food will bring you the health, happiness and security that you deeply desire. In truth, that which you seek through food can only be experienced when your choices serve the inner wisdom reflected by a purified Conscience.

Because food and the act of eating are so central to human culture, I often advise new students to begin their experimentation process in this particular "field of action." In fact, even Gandhi observed, "When you control your palate you can strengthen and vitalize the entire mind-body-sense complex." Does this mean that you can no longer eat the food you love? Not necessarily. It depends on which function of the mind is doing the "loving"—your powerful taste buds and the attachment you may have to certain kinds of food, or your purified Conscience.

Not long ago, while I was intently watching an episode of the popular *Diners, Drive-Ins, and Dives* television series, I was suddenly distracted by the rush of saliva filling my mouth as I witnessed people enjoying macaroni and cheese, hamburgers topped with French fried onion rings, and other familiar comfort foods. I must confess that for a vegetarian and a rather disciplined eater for more than 45 years, the experience was both shocking and instructive. First, I was astonished that my Senses and old, Unconscious habits were responding in such a juvenile, non-discriminating manner to the outrageously sensual prompts. Secondly, I felt an abiding compassion for other TV viewers who might not be armed with the tools provided in this book. I knew that if I were still a child—or an adult innocently handicapped by an untrained mind— I too would likely succumb to the call of my Senses, habit patterns and tide of the culture, just as I did when I was younger.

The truth is that since the human body is comprised of food and water, you are redefining yourself every time you bite off and swallow food. In fact, the personal philosophy you bring to this spiritually intimate relationship, and your attitude toward the entire miraculous process, reflects your concepts about every other relationship. Is it any wonder that changing eating habits is so challenging? If maintaining a well-balanced diet were solely a matter of making appropriate choices about nutrition, you might be a much healthier person than you are today. In practical terms, however, your eating habits are directly linked to powerful Unconscious emotional forces that seek happiness and security, and that tether you to your "family"— which I define here as the people with whom you regularly eat.

Imagine that after reading a few inspiring health articles, you told your closest friends and relatives you had decided to no longer eat the "Standard American Diet" that your family normally consumes. Instead, you announce that you will become a vegetarian. You will start eliminating flesh from your diet: no more poultry, pork, beef or fish (or anything else that has a face). At the same time, you will begin reducing or eliminating sugar, salt, unhealthy fats, simple carbs and alcohol. You can imagine how disturbed others would be. "Are you kidding? Are you no longer part of our group?" they'd wonder. "Are you rejecting our values, and us? Are we not worthy of your identification anymore?" *When you break with a group norm, your actions can be psychologically threatening to others, and their reactions can consciously or unconsciously pressure you to abandon your worthwhile intentions.* In situations like this your cheerfulness, kindness and reliable good sense of humor can enable you to speak your truth and hold your ground—all without causing unnecessary discomfort to others. This is exactly the kind of challenge a trained mind can help you with.

So how to begin? As with every experiment presented in this chapter, practice *ahimsa*—non-injury, non-harming. Understand that you are not alone. Changes like these are difficult for almost everyone, so be kind to yourself in every situation—even if you "fall off the wagon." The more you practice, the more skilled you will become at making better choices. So, metaphorically speaking, if you can't give up the whole cookie right now, try giving up half the cookie. The goal is to reduce your intake of the less-than-helpful food that your Senses and habits love, and to eat more of the food that loves you—*all* of you.

If that sounds like repression or denial of the "good life," I guarantee you it is just the opposite. Imagine for a moment that everything you've chosen to eat today is now benefitting the health and vitality of your blood vessels, eyes, joints, teeth, ears, skin, lymph system, thyroid, brain, muscles, heart, lungs, liver, bladder, spleen, intestines, gall bladder, stomach, kidneys, uterus and pancreas. And as a bonus, those choices are also providing you more flexibility, energy, optimism, creativity, improved elimination and lower health care costs. With all those positive benefits, would you still consider not eating a cheeseburger with bacon to be a denial of the "good life?"

Below are 16 specific suggestions. My recommendation is to try each experiment, one at a time, and commit to following that particular new suggestion for one week. Anybody can do anything for seven days! During the experiment, and at its conclusion, spend some time reflecting on the results. How do you feel? How comfortable is your digestion and elimination? How is your energy level? Was the quality of your sleep impacted? Have you noticed any change in your productivity? Nobody but you will know the answers to these questions.

As you experiment, continue to rely on your inner wisdom, reflected by your Conscience, when uncertainties arise. Have confidence that you are engaging in an important spiritual practice. Every time you heed the quiet voice of the Conscience and base your outer actions (in this case, what you choose to put into your body) on your Super Conscious Wisdom, you are building reserves of love, fearlessness and strength that you can access in other situations, as needed. Be aware that you are using the *Bridge of Yoga* as a tool to help guide your choices related to food. *After all, if you can't skillfully solve the problem of what's for dinner, how are you going to solve the great challenges of the world? Starting small builds critical skills.* At the conclusion of each week, you can decide if you want to adopt that particular new lifestyle choice into your toolbag of helpful, long-term habits.

### Experiments with Foods that Love You

1. Reduce or avoid sugar. Processed sugar and "high fructose corn syrup" are poison to your system. Don't bring sodas or sugar-laden baked goods home. Try natural alternative sweeteners like honey or stevia.

2. Avoid cold drinks during meals. According to Yoga Science cold liquids retard digestion and trigger the production of subtle substances that cause disease.

3. Chew your food well. Depending on the texture, chew 20-30 times before swallowing. You'll eat less, feel more satisfied, digest better, assimilate more completely and eliminate more easily.

4. Drink hot water. Drink 6-8 cups of plain hot water (the same temperature as coffee) every day. We call this the Million Dollar Prescription! It boosts energy and cleanses your entire urinary system.

5. Use mineral or sea salt. Refined table salt is chemically processed. Natural salts include trace minerals needed for a strong immune system.

6. Reduce or eliminate gluten. Gluten is an acknowledged inflammatory agent. Your brilliant, but delicate immune system and digestive tract will be grateful.

7. Eat quinoa as a grain substitute. It's alkalizing, relatively low in carbs and is a complete protein that provides all the essential amino acids.

8. Reduce or eliminate dairy. Proteins in dairy are very difficult to digest and lead to a host of digestive issues for many people.

9. Use ghee (clarified butter) instead of whole butter or margarine. It improves assimilation of nutrients and contains fewer undesirable solids.

10. Eat cilantro and basil to boost flavors and to cleanse the blood.

11. Eat a medley of three fresh vegetables daily. Use your favorites and change the trio often. A balance of colors ensures a spectrum of nutrients. Cook and garnish vegetables with garlic, herbs and olive oil.

12. Reduce or eliminate red meat, poultry, and fish. Flesh is highly acidic, lengthens stool transit time and taxes all digestive organs. We can be healthy and find other delicious sources of protein without taking a sentient life.

13. Eat fresh, first-generation foods daily. As often as possible, prepare food just before it is to be eaten. The life force contained in your food is greatly diminished in leftovers.

14. Take a pro-biotic supplement daily. This will help build healthy intestinal flora.

15. Leave a little space in your stomach at the end of each meal. That space improves digestive efficiency.

16. As appropriate, add a vitamin D supplement to your diet to enhance the body's immune response.

### Experiment 2
### Lies Versus Truth

To lie or not to lie, that is the question. The internal dialogue that takes place while we decide whether or not to serve the higher Truth usually sounds like this: "If I lie, the outcome I fear will probably just disappear. But if I speak what I think is true, the outcome I fear is going to cause me pain." That's how most human beings struggle with the Ego's desire for short-term, limited gratification versus the long-term benefit offered by heeding the Conscience. It's the age-old conversation between the devil on one shoulder and the angel on the other.

But the simple Truth is that a lie cannot save us from a painful consequence. Any action against the wisdom of the Conscience will eventually lead to some physical, mental, emotional or spiritual dis-ease or pain. And if we do not heed the message of pain at a low decibel level, the message will simply get louder and louder until dis-ease becomes full-blown disease.

If the Truth be told, most of us lie—and we might even do it every day. It's not an attractive part of our humanity, but if we're absolutely honest with ourselves, we must admit that lying appears to be an integral part of being human. We all serve non-Truth in certain kinds of situations, wittingly or unwittingly, by intentionally making statements for the purpose of deception. This tendency is worthy of our investigation.

Why do we lie and cause so much pain and suffering to ourselves and others? Since we already have a Conscience that can discriminate between the Truth and non-Truth, why aren't we hard-wired from birth to use the Conscience to serve only the Truth and to be free, happy, healthy and secure? What power motivates us to lie, even against our better judgment—almost as if forcing us? My personal experiments with Truth indicate that the primary cause of our lying is the Ego's excessive attachment to self-preservation. *It lives in the form of subtle fears that hide below the surface level of the conscious mind.*

What is it that triggers the Ego's belief that someone or something is dangerous, likely to cause pain, and that a lie might protect us? In many cases, the simple answer is ignorance. The Ego has learned to ignore the Truth that we are citizens of two worlds and that our subtle-most core is an eternal ocean of consciousness, wisdom and bliss (a.k.a. God). Instead, the Ego mistakenly defines the concepts "I," "me" and "mine" exclusively as the body and the personality. The Ego doesn't know about your Essential Nature or the hidden treasure, your Super Conscious Wisdom.

By relying exclusively on the inherent limitations of the Ego, Senses and Unconscious Mind, each of us has grown up from birth under a grand illusion that motivates us to lie in a vain attempt to obliterate fear. Every day we innocently accept the false, egoic, family and cultural suggestions that "I" am a separate individual. Religionists even have a name for this condition. They call it "original sin," as if there were nothing we could do to end our ignorance. In fact, the concept of "sin" is so identified with punishment, pain and eternal damnation that we have forgotten that the word "sin" came into the English language from its origin as a Greek archery term. It simply meant that an archer had "missed the intended target." We need not condemn ourselves to the pain associated with the cultural concept of sin. Instead, we can contemplate the factors that brought about the error in our aim, and thus gain the clarity and wisdom to redirect the flight of our next arrow. In the process we'll learn how to transform the "hell" of guilt and fear into the "heaven" of self-confidence and comfort.

Are you ready to go beyond the fears that cause the pain of serving non-Truth? If so, here are five essential rules that have helped me in my own personal practice of experimenting with the Truth. As you uncover and employ the Truth, your improved vision will change your consciousness—and that of the planet.

1. The Truth must always be in harmony with *ahimsa* (non-injury, non-harming, non-violence), the highest principle of Yoga Science. If what you believe to be true is in

conflict with *ahimsa*, it must be relegated to the lower status of a mere fact, not the Truth. Please remember that facts that cause injury are not to be served in speech or action. If you feel you must speak a fact that can cause injury to another human being, dive deep into the ocean of consciousness and you will find different, kinder words to use. This conscious process enables you to serve your own truth without injury to others or repression to yourself.

2. Consider your own mind-body-sense complex to be your personal laboratory for experiments with the Truth. This scientific perspective will become your trustworthy technique for finding and knowing what is to be done.

3. In searching for Truth, coordinate the Four Functions of the Mind, and then heed the counsel of the Conscience, for it alone can reflect Truth into your conscious mind.

4. Recognize that fear always manifests in one of two ways: the fear I won't get what I want, and the fear I might lose what I have.

5. Remember to employ your will power to serve Truth and sacrifice the Ego's attachment to the non-Truth.

### Experiment 3
### Use the Breath to Quiet the Mind

The Psalms inform us that "Each human life is but a breath." Without breath, our lives would be impossible. The exchange of oxygen for carbon dioxide in the lungs is certainly essential for the human being to function, but Yoga Science states that air is not what animates the city of life. Rather, our lives are sustained by an extremely powerful form of subtle energy known as *prana* that accompanies the air we breathe. On the most subtle level, it is the vital *prana* that animates the mind-body-sense complex. If, for instance, you were to force air into the lungs of a cadaver it would not get up and walk away. Why is that? Because it is *prana*, already present in a living body, that invites, receives and distributes the life force of *prana* carried on the vehicle of breath. It is *prana* alone, not the mediums of air, food, or water, that enlivens the body and mind.

Breathing exercises, known as *pranayama* in Sanskrit, are one of the tools you have as a Yoga Scientist to calm and focus your mind. *Pranayama* is a compound word. It is a combination of the word *prana*, meaning energy, and *yama*, which means control. The quality and state of your breath is in fact a barometer that indicates the state of your mind. As you undertake the experiments below, it is especially important to practice *ahimsa*—non-injury, non-harming. No attempt to control or regulate the breath should ever cause you stress or anxiety, or cause any jerks or irregularities in the breath. If it does, abandon the technique and just quietly observe your breath without trying to change it. The simple act of becoming aware of your breath can yield powerful results in the mind. Also, never extend the breath beyond your comfortable capacity by inhaling or exhaling as much air as possible. With continued practice, your capacity will naturally increase, but this cannot be rushed.

There is an entire science behind the practice of *pranayama*, and there are numerous advanced techniques that you may want to learn eventually. In the beginning, however, if you just remember to keep your breath "smooth and comfortable" as you experiment, you will reap the rewards.

### Diaphragmatic Breathing
The diaphragmatic breathing technique is one of the most powerful tools you have to quiet the body and the mind, and it is available to you 24 hours a day, 7 days a week, 365 days a year. If you watch a newborn baby

## How Diaphragmatic Breathing Works

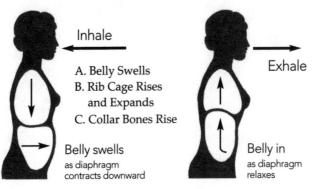

Inhale

A. Belly Swells
B. Rib Cage Rises
   and Expands
C. Collar Bones Rise

Belly swells
as diaphragm
contracts downward

Exhale

Belly in
as diaphragm
relaxes

breathe, you will notice the baby naturally using the abdomen while breathing diaphragmatically. Your goal is simply to re-establish the body's innate respiratory pattern—not by breathing from the upper chest, which is an unhealthy, acquired habit, but rather, by consciously employing the diaphragm, one of the body's strongest muscles, in your breathing process. Ideally, with continued practice, diaphragmatic breathing will once again become your "default" breath, like it was when you were a baby, providing ongoing benefits to your body (especially your over-taxed nervous system) and your mind.

### Crocodile Posture

The Crocodile Posture is an excellent way to become reacquainted with diaphragmatic breathing. That's because when you are in this posture you automatically have to breathe diaphragmatically. Before you assume the Crocodile Posture, make sure you're wearing clothing that fits loosely around your waist. If you wear eyeglasses, take them off, and put them in a safe place. Lie face down on your stomach on the floor, positioning your feet a little wider than shoulder width apart. Your toes may turn in

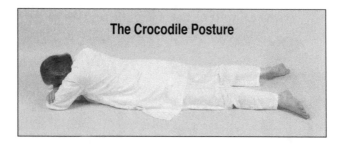

**The Crocodile Posture**

or out. Crossing your arms in front of your body, clasp the right hand around the left bicep, just above the left elbow. Then clasp the left hand around the right bicep, just above the right elbow. Rest your forehead on your forearm, just above the wrist.

Don't position your arms too far out in front of you, which would bring the chest flush with the floor. Neither should you position the arms too close to the chest, which would put undue stress on the lower back and pinch the neck muscles. The ideal is to create a slight curve in the lower back, but without any strain.

Once you have established the Crocodile Posture, begin to focus your awareness on your breath at the belly, or navel region. Your breath should be full, but not beyond your normal, comfortable capacity. If it is helpful to you, imagine that a balloon is positioned in the belly, just behind the navel. With each inhalation, the balloon will inflate and the belly will swell, and with each exhalation the balloon will deflate, and the belly will gently contract. If you have correctly established the Crocodile Posture, you will automatically be breathing diaphragmatically. As you inhale, you will notice the belly swelling gently—pressing against the floor. As this occurs, the ribcage rises and expands, and the collar bones move upward. As you exhale, the belly contracts slightly, as the imagined balloon is deflating.

Practice diaphragmatic breathing for five minutes at least once a day in the Crocodile Posture. When you are ready to get up, gently turn onto your right side and rest for a few seconds. Then, push off with your left hand into a sitting position. Pause again for one full breath before rising to a standing position.

### The Vagus Nerve

A quick anatomy lesson will help you fully understand the value of the Crocodile Posture and diaphragmatic breathing. The diaphragm, in its resting state, is a large muscle that resembles the dome of an open parachute. It separates the chest cavity (containing your heart and lungs) from the abdominal cavity that holds the organs of the digestive, urinary, and reproductive systems. Running directly through the diaphragm into the abdominal cavity is the vagus nerve, which extends all the way from your brain. The vagus nerve is the longest cranial nerve in the body, and it is responsible for regulating the "fight-flight-freeze" response whenever you encounter a real or imagined threat—whether it be a saber tooth tiger like our ancestors faced, or any number of hypothetical situations that you fear might arise. Once the threat has passed, the vagus nerve—reassured by the gentle, massaging movement of the diaphragm—signals the brain that the body can return to its pre-stressed condition: the heart rate can slow down, saliva and digestive processes can go back to normal, and the breath can lengthen.

But this ideal functioning does not regularly occur in our modern world because most of us breathe primarily in our upper chest, and there is very little, if any, movement in the diaphragm. As a result, the brain never gets the message from the vagus nerve that the body can calm down. It is only through diaphragmatic breathing that the vagus nerve can be massaged and stimulated, and convinced sufficiently to tell the brain that the danger has passed; that the body and mind can return to (or remain in) a state of relaxed equilibrium. *This is a physiological response that you can activate at will.* Full and even diaphragmatic breathing also massages the internal organs. This rhythmic motion transmits beneficial messages to the entire autonomic nervous system, messages that encourage all the bodily systems to operate optimally.

### One-Minute Breath Meditation

This one-minute meditation on the breath is an easy-to-do and effective practice that can be helpful in almost any situation. Regardless of whether you are seated or standing, simply attend to both the inhalation and exhalation of your breath, for 60 seconds, at the bridge between the two nostrils—where the nostrils meet the upper lip. Focus all of your attention there at that one location. Even if you are at work and cannot sit in privacy or close your eyes, the benefits of this practice will be profound. During this practice distractions may appear. Just acknowledge any distraction, let it go without anger or judgment, and return your attention back to the breath. This short breath-awareness meditation will calm your mind, center your attention, give you access to your reserves of energy and send wonderfully beneficial and reassuring messages to the entire autonomic nervous system. At the end of one minute, you may decide to extend the meditation for a second minute, or conclude the practice.

### Experiment 4
### Strengthening Relationships

I often ask my students: Do you desire to experience loving, meaningful and richly rewarding relationships? Is it important for you to be happy and content? Do you want to reduce or eliminate the various forms of dis-ease in your life? Almost universally, the answer is a resounding "Yes!" If this is true for you, you can achieve everything you earnestly desire by honestly examining the ways you deal with relationships.

Just for a moment, stop and think about the wide variety of relationships you have every day. Think of your spouse (or boyfriend / girlfriend / partner / lover). Think of your child, parents, siblings, friends, extended family, neighbors, pets, the people you work for or with, and those you do business with (like the banker, supermarket cashier, auto mechanic, waitress, teacher, or doctor). Now, consider your more remote relationships with your local, state and national government officials, and all the celebrity types you know through television, radio, films, recordings, and social media. Then add the thousands of intimate relationships you have with your own body, the food you eat, your breath, your Senses, as well as your mind and its many thoughts, desires, memories, imaginations, emotions and concepts. Let's face it, you have a lot of relationships!

Every single relationship requires you to take some kind of action. Essentially, that is what having a relationship means. When you have a relationship, it means that a thought, desire, or emotion is commanding your attention and requiring you to respond. Relationships imply action just as action implies a relationship, and your choice of which thoughts to think, which words to speak, and which actions to take will determine whether your relationships bring you happiness, or sorrow.

Now look more closely at a certain category of relationships that have an out-sized impact on each of us—the people we interact with every day at home or at work. Sometimes it feels like the most challenging relationships we have are with the people we care for most. Perhaps this is because rather than seeing them and loving them for who they are, we are actually loving *our pre-conceived idea* of them. And when they say or do things that don't match *our idea* of what they should say or do, we feel disappointed, betrayed or angry. Imagine for a moment that someone you love feels the same way about the things you say or do.

The truth is, of course, that the same Super Conscious Wisdom that fills your heart and mind also fills theirs. Just like it fills mine. Your Essential Nature—*Sat-Chit-Ananda*—is also their Essential Nature. Even if they do not (yet) realize it. Even if they have not read this book. Even if they have different political beliefs than you. Or different tastes in movies or food. Or different habits related to exercise or work. When we begin to understand that each and every one of us has access to the same source of Divine Love, our compassion for one another grows exponentially. We become more considerate and loving when we let the Conscience guide us in relating to one another at this higher level. Creative solutions arise to solve problems that may have plagued our relationships for years.

It may seem obvious, but it is worth pausing to consider that the quality of your relationships can—and will—suffer if you don't give them your attention. As I say when I lead my students in meditation, *"Attention is Love."* Your Conscience knows this and will guide you toward making decisions that cultivate happier, healthier relationships and increase your capacity to give and receive love. Your task is to listen for the quiet voice of the Conscience when you engage in relationships with those around you.

My advice is to begin experimenting with those closest to you, the people you see every day. After you complete each experiment, reflect on how you feel. Did you experience any anxiety, anger, or fear? How did you benefit from the experience? Evaluate how you feel physically, mentally, emotionally and spiritually. Regardless of the outcome, congratulate yourself on doing the experiment, and know that the more frequently you base your thoughts, words and deeds on your own inner wisdom, the more fulfilling all your relationships will become— even those that previously have been challenging.

### Listen to Others
When you're talking with someone, give them your full, complete and undivided attention. Avoid interrupting. Put your phone down. When they are finished speaking, recap what the other person has said. Let them know they were heard, even if your Ego disliked or was bored with what was said. Offering your attention to another person is one of the greatest gifts you can give.

### Practice Patience
When you find yourself getting impatient or bored with another person, ask your Conscience to guide you toward understanding and love rather than avoidance or anger. Try setting aside your own personal needs, and put another person's needs first (just as an experiment).

### Observe Anger
When you become aware of anger, take a time out. Don't allow negative emotion to poison your entire body. Pause to examine which function of the mind authored the anger, and ask your Conscience if there is a more compassionate, non-injurious way to express what you truly need in this situation. Listen to the wise and good counsel of the Conscience when you re-engage with the person or situation that triggered your anger.

### Give Love Freely
When you find yourself withholding love, ask the Conscience, your *Buddhi*, if building a wall to protect yourself is in everyone's best interest. If not, reach out to the

other person—without expectation. Your Conscience will help you know how and when to reach out.

## Experiment 5
## Preparing to Receive Sleep

The enjoyment and satisfaction provided by sleep are higher than those provided by any other pleasures, even food and sex. In sleep the body rests and repairs itself. It is important to realize that we are more likely to have a deep, restful sleep if we resolve every choice during the day by following the advice of the Conscience. Such diverse choices could include: attention to *ahimsa* in all our relationships, eating our biggest meal at midday, relaxing the body and mind through simple stretching exercises like yoga, and practicing diaphragmatic breathing throughout the day. When it is difficult to sleep, or when we awake in the morning feeling tired, it's often because we have anxieties about issues left unresolved at the end of the day. Your grandmother was right: don't go to bed angry!

The following experiments will help to prepare your body and mind to receive deep, restful and healing sleep. As with the experiments related to food and eating, I suggest that you try each experiment one at a time for the duration of a week and keep a journal to record your observations.

1. Go to bed before 10:00p.m. This will allow your body to take advantage of the natural healing that occurs between the hours of 10:00p.m. and 2:00a.m. and will prepare you to rise with the sun.

2. Set a cut-off time for all electronic devices at least one hour before bedtime—no phones, computers, emails or television.

3. Don't eat anything within two to three hours of going to bed. Experiment with eating your largest meal at midday, rather than at the traditional dinner time.

4. Go to bed and wake up at the same time every day. A regular schedule will signal to your body and mind when it is time to rest and when it is time to act.

5. Pay attention to what you do immediately before closing your eyes. Consider reading an inspirational passage or jotting down something you are grateful for that happened during the course of the day. These moments will impact the activity of your Unconscious mind while you sleep.

## Experiment 6
## One-Pointed Attention

*The mind is a mischief-maker.*
*It jumps from doubt to doubt; it puts obstacles in the way.*
*It weaves a net and gets entangled in it.*
*It is ever discontented; it runs after a hundred things*
*and away from another hundred.*

SATYA SAI BABA

The prevailing tide of our culture encourages multi-pointed attention. Today each of us is encouraged to multi-task, to be like a short-order cook and fry the eggs, toast the bread, brew the coffee and serve everything simultaneously and on time—without breaking yolks, burning toast or serving coffee that's less than piping hot. Then it's immediately on to the next order and the next. It's no longer enough merely to be good at what you do. People are urged to develop expertise in many different areas—and are often asked to report to more than one boss during the workday.

The overwhelming influence of the smart phone has added to this new multi-focused normal. How often do you pull out your phone to check your social media feed or Google something while you're engaged in face-to-face conversation? How often does the alert of a new text, tweet, email, Instagram story, or Facebook post pull your attention away from whatever you are attempting to do? Indeed, these small and powerful hand-held devices represent an imposing threat to our ability to stay focused. It must be said, however, that our own minds are infinitely more powerful than this technology. For our health and well-being, we must endeavor to take back our control.

Performing more than one task at the same time may seem like an efficient use of energy, but this habit takes a significant toll on your health. Recent scientific studies conclude that multitasking asks the brain to function beyond its capacity. The brain simply cannot process more than one piece of information at a time. It might appear that you can drive and talk on the cell phone simultaneously, but to accomplish both, the brain has to run back and forth between the two activities. When faced with the demands of multitasking, the brain actually becomes overloaded, slows down and sends an S.O.S. to the adrenals to release stress hormones into the body. Prolonged release of adrenaline eventually leads to sleep deprivation, a depressed immune system, anxiety, burnout and depression.

The demands of the culture and its omnipresent technology are quite opposed to the single-pointed attention that we cultivate through the practice of Yoga Science. When your mind is one-pointed, you have access to the unlimited wisdom and creativity at the center of your being. The greatest artistic, innovative and productive achievements in history have been facilitated through minds exercising one-pointed attention. Similarly, at the pinnacle of any Olympic competition, the gold medal is won by the athlete whose mind has been made one-pointed. The gold medalist possesses the skill to remain focused regardless of competitive thoughts, desires or emotions that could steal energy and attention.

Never undervalue the power of your own attention! Attention means love, and love increases interest in the object of your attention. To thoroughly know anything, to discover or create anything, you must give your heart to it—which means your attention. The greater the focus of attention, the more profound the blessing.

The key to contentment lies in understanding that although we have little or no control over the thoughts that come to us, we always have a say over whether or not we continue to give them the attention that will empower them to shape the events and relationships of our lives. As the Compassionate Buddha taught, "You are what you think." What you think today will determine what you experience tomorrow.

### The Laser and the Soaker Hose

Laser technology provides an apt analogy to illustrate the benefits of concentrating our attention. The elementary unit of light energy is called a photon. Incandescent, fluorescent and LED bulbs are designed to produce ambient light by scattering photons in many directions, bouncing them off the ceiling, walls and floor. This disorganized light energy serves to illuminate low-light environments. By directing all the photons in one direction simultaneously, however, scientists create a laser beam powerful enough to cut through steel and precise enough to perform micro-surgery.

When you learn to cultivate one-pointed attention, you apply the principle of laser technology to the energy field of the mind and produce similarly profound results.

Learning to focus your entire attention (mental energy) toward a single point enables you to expand your consciousness by tapping into the library of intuitive wisdom within you.

If the laser beam is an example of one-pointed attention, the soaker hose is an equally apt example of multi-pointed attention. A soaker hose is like an ordinary garden hose with one small but critical difference: a multitude of tiny holes allows water to escape all along the fifty or so feet of its length. This provides gentle irrigation for plants and shrubs, but because the force of the water is dissipated along its length, there's very little water pressure at the far end.

Just like a soaker hose, the untrained mind dissipates a tremendous amount of creative energy by indulging a host of little desires and entertaining a legion of habitual thoughts. If you're in the habit of multitasking, you're likely to find yourself with inadequate supplies of energy, will power and creative ideas when life makes an important demand.

Now, imagine taking a roll of duct tape and carefully sealing all the holes along the length of the soaker hose of your mind. Closing those countless outlets will give you a tremendous force of energy with which to work. When you learn to conserve and transform the energy of the small, petty desires of *preya* (including the tireless calls of the Senses,) you'll have access to endless healing energy, will power and creativity.

Certain relationships that require an action may seem insignificant, yet they can be powerful opportunities to bring you closer to fulfillment—if you can practice one-pointed attention. The following experiments represent small steps that will help you train your mind and focus your attention. Try them and record the results in your journal.

## Experiments to Focus Your
## ONE-POINTED ATTENTION

### Pay Attention While Eating

How often do you engage in a secondary activity while you are eating? It might be watching television, reading, or talking on the phone. By doing two activities at the same time (multitasking), you're training the mind to divide its attention. As a consequence, your body will neither digest as thoroughly nor assimilate the nutrition of the food as completely as it could if you were mindfully eating with one-pointed attention (monotasking). Furthermore, you simply cannot fully enjoy the pleasures of the flavor, texture, scent and colors of your food while half of your attention is devoted to the evening news. Experiment by turning off the television, closing your book, and putting down your phone when it is time to eat. Focus your attention on the food you are ingesting. Chew slowly and completely. Recognize that the food you put into your body will be converted to energy. Be grateful every time you have the opportunity to eat.

### Focus at Work or School

The training of attention can continue in all your activities. For instance, when you're at work trying to complete a task and the phone rings, you may have a great desire to continue what you're doing while you talk on the phone. "I can do both," you tell yourself. "This conversation is not particularly demanding." It's probably true that you could accomplish both tasks—at less than full efficiency, but I urge you to experiment.

As a Yoga Scientist, ask the Conscience which desire represents the *preya* and which is the *shreya*. If the telephone call is the *shreya*, try to witness and surrender the desire to continue working, then give one hundred percent of your attention to your conversation. Place your pen on your desk, take your fingers off the keyboard, and direct your complete and undivided attention to the person who wants to speak with you. No one else will ever know the mental deliberation you've made, but by exercising this kind of detachment and discrimination, you'll develop a sharp focus of your mind for the benefit of every upcoming relationship.

### Do Your Chores Mindfully

Most of us engage in regular chores like cooking, washing dishes, and doing laundry in order to keep our lives running smoothly. Use these daily chores as opportunities to focus your attention. If you're chopping vegetables, pay close attention as the knife slices through each piece. When washing the dishes, don't entertain distracting or annoying thoughts. Instead, give your attention to the sensual pleasure of immersing your hands in warm, sudsy water. Watch mindfully as the soft, wet sponge caresses the smooth porcelain, and the newly sparkling glassware catches the light. You'll find that you might actually enjoy the experience. When doing laundry, pay attention to how you handle the clothes. Enjoy the warmth as you pull the clothes from the dryer. Fold each article of clothing carefully and lovingly. Every activity, completed with full attention, will be more pleasurable and rewarding—added benefits as you skillfully hone your one-pointed concentration.

FINALLY, I want to emphasize again that I am not asking you to blindly believe anything presented in this book. Instead, I simply ask that you trust your Conscience—at least enough to begin to experiment. The experiments offered in this chapter present an opportunity. As you conclude each one, put on your "Doubting

Thomas" hat, and objectively ask yourself, "Do I feel better—physically, mentally, emotionally and spiritually?" I'm betting that, like me, you too will answer, "Yes, I do feel better."

As you engage in this process, some experiments will be more easily mastered than others. Some may feel very difficult at first. And hopefully, you'll create your own experiments as well. Regardless, I promise you that your sincere effort will not go unrewarded. Each time you succeed, you will be building your will power, which will enable you to succeed in the *next* experiment. You can do this. You just have to commit wholeheartedly to trying.

CHAPTER 7

# *Where to Start if You Don't Know Where to Start*

*Waking up to who you are requires*
*letting go of who you imagine yourself to be.*

ALAN WATTS

If you are curious enough to try *something*, but you can't quite wrap your head around eliminating sugar, or turning off the TV while you eat, it's okay. I understand. Our habit patterns run deep. And the older we are, the deeper they run, those channels in our Unconscious mind.

I am convinced, however, that each one of us is intimately familiar with the function of the mind that we call *Buddhi*—the Conscience. I believe that we *know* when we are following the wisdom of our purified Conscience. When we make a skillful choice regarding what we eat, we *know*. When we are kind to other people, we *know*. When we spread love rather than fear or anger, we *know*.

And when we do the opposite, we also know.

One of the ways we know we have acted skillfully is that we feel better—whether it is physically, mentally, emotionally, or spiritually. How do you feel after you eat a fresh, wholesome lunch? How about after a double hamburger, fries and a soda? How do you feel when you volunteer your time in service to others? How about after a Saturday afternoon spent channel surfing while lying on the sofa? You know. We all know.

Here are a few suggestions for those among us who genuinely want to make a change, but are also genuinely not sure how to begin. Try one of these experiments for a day, then decide if you want to extend the period to a week. After a week, you can decide if you want to try another experiment. Don't think of it as a New Year's resolution; it's just a simple experiment. It might even be fun! You're just indulging your curiosity. You're a budding Yoga Scientist at work. Nothing more, nothing less.

Each time you experiment with making a wise choice by tapping into your Super Conscious Wisdom, you are purifying the Conscience. Over time, and with continued experimentation, it will become easier to hear the quiet but certain voice of the Conscience. Each time you make a skillful choice, you are building strength and resolve that will help you make other skillful choices about issues that might not be quite as obvious. You're in training. We all are. The important thing is to start somewhere. Let your Conscience be your guide!

### A Beginner's Menu of Experiments

1. Eat and drink less of the stuff you already know is not nourishing. If you can't give up a whole cookie today, try eating only half a cookie—just for the sake of the experiment. If you can't give up potato chips, try limiting how often you eat them, or how many you eat. Use whatever method works for you to start to change your habits. Be intentional about it.

2. Make your bed every day. This small act has a surprisingly positive impact that lasts all day, all the way up to and including when we go back to bed.

3. Drink hot water during the day instead of coffee, tea, or soda. You can microwave it or heat it on the stove or use an electric kettle. Try to drink at least one more cup of hot water a day than you are drinking right now. Work your way up to 6-8 cups of hot water daily.

4. Experiment with stepping away from your phone for an hour every day. You could try this while you are working or while you are eating. Is there a difference if you can still see the phone (even if it is not within reach) compared to what happens when you physically remove it from the room? Also, experiment by charging your phone overnight someplace other than your bedroom.

5. Try to stop interrupting people so often. We all do it, sometimes just because we're excited to express our enthusiastic agreement. Practice listening patiently while family members or colleagues attempt to communicate. Notice the impact this has on people. Notice how you feel when you are permitted to finish your thoughts without interruption. When you catch yourself interrupting someone, stop and apologize, then let them finish expressing their thought. This takes practice, but it is worth the effort.

6. Before you engage in a difficult conversation, pause and breathe diaphragmatically. You could take five breaths. If you don't have time for this because the person is standing right in front of you, you can always take one deep breath before speaking. Notice how that one breath changes the energy between you and the other person.

7. Choose one small daily chore, and when you perform that chore, give it your full attention. When you

notice that your mind has wandered away from what you are doing, gently bring it back. Try this experiment with something very simple like brushing your teeth.

8. When you recognize that you are worrying about something, simply notice. Acknowledge that it is really only the personality doing the worrying. Take note of the worrying, and just consider the possibility that you could do something different with that energy. You may go back to worrying, but just for a moment acknowledge that it's really only the personality worrying. Not the real *you*. That recognition in itself is a big step in learning detachment.

9. Whatever that one thing is you do that you know you should stop—try stopping it, just for today. And whatever that one thing is you don't do that you *know* you should start—try starting it, just for today. Take one small step today, without concern for what will happen tomorrow.

10. Practice smiling. The sages tell us that cheerfulness is the most powerful mantra. Look for one extra opportunity to smile every day, even if you are just smiling to yourself in the mirror.

# *Afterword:*
# *Self-Reliance and Response-Ability*
# *in a Modern Age*

*Life is like a piano.*
*What you get out of it depends on how you play it.*

ALBERT EINSTEIN

Hindsight is 20/20. Many of us have heard this adage our entire lives. It makes sense. When we look back at a situation after some time has passed, we are often able to see things more clearly than we could when we were "in the moment." As Yoga Scientists, our goal is to cultivate that clarity of vision in *every* moment. We accomplish this by relying on the Conscience to access our Super Conscious Wisdom in all our relationships.

The collective pain that so many in America have experienced in the first two decades of the 21st century, starting with the attack on the World Trade Center on September 11, 2001 and culminating with the global coronavirus pandemic of 2020, may, in fact, represent the greatest opportunity for individual and collective growth that we have seen in generations.

According to a poll conducted in early 2020 by *The Wall Street Journal* and NBC News (before COVID-19 fully displayed its power), approximately 80% of Americans surveyed said they believed the country was "out of control." Read that statistic again—eight out of ten people felt their country was *out of control*. America is a country with a long history of political division, but in the year 2020, the divide felt deeper and wider, and potentially far more dangerous than it had since the Civil War.

Regardless of political affiliation, every citizen in our great nation faced the relentless politicization of major circumstances that threatened the viability of our government, our occupations, and our very lives. These events included two impeachments of a President, the loss of tens of millions of jobs and more than half a million lives due to the pandemic, a fraught and contested national election, and ongoing, even violent, national protests that demanded a thorough re-imagining of what it means, for each of us, to be human beings.

This kind of polarized environment takes a major toll on the well-being of every citizen. CBS News reported that in 2019, more than 20 percent of Americans had symptoms of depression or anxiety. By early June 2020, however, researchers estimated that percentage had tripled. *Nearly two-thirds of all Americans were suffering acutely, on a daily basis.* And I believe that was a low estimate.

But depression and anxiety aren't the only challenges we face. I'll name just a few. Let these symptoms wash over your consciousness, and feel how familiar they are to you: anger, agitation, anguish, apprehension, consternation, desperation, discomfort, fear, foreboding, franticness, misgiving, nervousness, panic, rage, tension, terror, torment, uncertainty, unease, and worry. All sobering, to say the least.

It is important to note that these trials came on the heels of some of the most tumultuous years in modern memory. No wonder so many people felt things were out of control. Harrowing, infuriating stories emerged from the #MeToo movement. The opioid crisis continues to bring pain and ruin to great swaths of our country. Wildfires, hurricanes, and other disasters have displaced many and caused terrible loss. Mass shootings at schools have become so commonplace that children are familiar with the phrase "active shooter," and know what to do if they encounter one. Imagine what this does to a child's mind. If you are a teenager, you are all too familiar with this reality.

Intensely aware of these reactions in the country, I've been contemplating what it would take to turn things around. At this point in human history, what changes, if any, could this present generation make that would profoundly benefit the collective good? Somewhere in this contemplation process an amusing 1955 Frank Sinatra novelty song that provides a surprisingly important hidden meaning popped into my mind. Written by four-time Academy Award winning lyricist Sammy Cahn, the words to "Love and Marriage" go like this:

Love and marriage, love and marriage,
Go together like a horse and carriage.
This I tell ya, brother,
you can't have one without the other.

Love and marriage, love and marriage,
It's an institute you can't disparage.
Ask the local gentry and they will say
it's elementary.

Try, try, try to separate them, it's an illusion.
Try, try, try and you only come to this conclusion:

Love and marriage, love and marriage,
Go together like a horse and carriage.
Dad was told by mother you can't have one,
You can't have none,
You can't have one—without the other.

I had no idea why that song from my childhood appeared. Was it just some nonsensical trump card my Ego was playing? It certainly didn't seem to advance my understanding of how we might achieve a more perfect union. And I couldn't imagine how it could possibly hasten the success of the coronavirus vaccine, put people back to work, or help resolve the uncivil and often poisonous political environment. But regardless, the song continued. And as more time went by, the verse's hypnotic musical hook just kept repeating and repeating in my mind. Love and marriage, love and marriage, Go together like a horse and carriage. Love and marriage, love and marriage, Go together like a horse and carriage.

Then, suddenly, it hit me—in the form of a question. "What two concepts," I asked myself, "am I personally familiar with today that might, if linked together, lead to a reduction, and possibly an elimination of all the many challenges we now face?"

And as soon as I was able to posit that question, the answer came—as if the question and answer were two sides of the same coin.

The two-fold answer I could now "see" was a pair of misunderstood, but vital, life-enhancing concepts: "Self-Reliance" and "Response-Ability." As you'll notice, both are compound words. For the Yoga Scientist, the concept "Self-Reliance" couples our divine, higher Self with reliance, and "Response-Ability" reflects a revised understanding of the word responsibility: namely, the ability to respond. As we learn to rely more and more on the Super

Conscious Wisdom at the core of our being, we will definitely attain the ability to respond skillfully and rewardingly with each of our thoughts, words and deeds. All of a sudden it seemed so obvious—this pair of concepts is all we need. Hammer and nail. Peanut butter and jelly. Hand and glove. Love and marriage. And here's how I know it's possible.

### "Self-Reliance"

In 1989 my wife Jenness and I traveled to California to visit one of our dearest teachers and colleagues, Eknath Easwaran. While with him, I explained that Yoga Science had become the guiding force in our lives, but we still worried about money. It seemed to us, I told him, that this philosophy and science would work best for people certain of receiving a paycheck every week, health insurance and a pension. We, on the other hand, were self-employed. The fact that Jenness was a painter and I was an art dealer meant that we never knew from one day to the next if we would have enough money to pay our bills. So we asked for some advice.

Without hesitation, and with a loving twinkle in his eye that I still recall to this day, Easwaran responded, "Your problem is this: you consider yourself self-employed. *I am employed by the Self.*" Hearing that one turn of phrase, we both recognized that the antidote for all our worries could be found by earnestly practicing Yoga Science.

Easwaran's reply taught us that the physical, mental and emotional pain we suffered by worrying was a direct consequence of being enslaved to the limited, often faulty, perspectives of the personality. To end our dis-ease, we knew we had to begin viewing relationships from a "higher" perspective—and that meant we had to expand our sense of "I-ness." As newly hired employees of the "Higher" Self, we set out to consciously identify and set aside longstanding, powerful and unhealthy habits by relying exclusively on the Divine wisdom of the mind's Conscience for every decision.

Once we made the decision to willingly convert our mind-body-sense complexes into our personal laboratories for conducting Yoga Science experiments, the universe immediately and lovingly responded by beginning to reveal the profound wisdom of Yoga Psychology. This system is both practical and helpful, and is presented to you in the pages of this book. It introduced us to the Four Functions of the Mind. It taught us how the mind operates, and how to train the mind to become more efficient, reliable and wise—enhancing its ability to make conscious, discriminating choices in every relationship.

Through our own personal experience we discovered that the science of Yoga is not just a scholarly pursuit. It is a moment-by-moment and thought-by-thought guide for living. Our path became clear. In order to end our distress, we simply had to become loyal employees—of the higher Self. This in no way meant repression or giving in to unhelpful and injurious Unconscious concepts. Rather, it implied welcoming, witnessing and honoring faulty concepts and then consciously sacrificing them—so that they were powerless to control our actions.

### "Response-Ability"

As Jenness and I became more comfortable with the notion that we are essentially spiritual beings—*Sat-Chit-Ananda*—living in the material world, something extraordinary began to happen. Our loyalty to the Self, our "Self-Reliance," had a profound impact on our ability to respond creatively in every situation. When we let go of our dependence on the faulty concepts of an unruly and untrained mind, we became more perceptive and creative. We were no longer triggered by the same things that had once tripped us up.

This detached perspective effectively created an enlarged space between the stimulus of a thought and our eventual response to that thought. The space between stimulus and response automatically provided us real freedom in every situation. That liberty made it easier to calm our minds, to hear the wise and good counsel of the Conscience, and to employ the necessary will power, so that our ultimate response would be in alignment with the Super Conscious Wisdom of the higher Self.

Let's look again at why this might seem to be so difficult to do. For several reasons, human birth presents an ongoing, unimaginably challenging assignment—one that can severely test our capacity to be responsible. First, nobody explained to us that there exists a critically important relationship between the mind and the body. It took me decades to find out that the mind determines how and when the body moves in the world—and that includes everything we think, say and do. This is wisdom I trust you have begun to understand through your sincere reflection and experimentation with what has been presented to you in this book.

Second, with all the years of schooling we had to go through, we were never provided a qualified teacher to properly instruct us on how the mind/body relationship operates, and what, if anything, we're required to do every minute of every day to assure that the entire system works efficiently and rewardingly. Third, as you now know, every bodily action—including every thought, word and deed—is followed by a specific consequence that leads us eventually to either fulfillment or to some form of physical, mental or emotional pain. The Law of Karma wasn't taught in any of my public education classrooms!

Yet here we are. Yoga Science has offered us a framework to understand that the mind is not one monolithic decision-making machine. In actuality, the mind, in its present, unattended-to condition, often exhibits a dangerous state of anarchy and inner conflict among its four separate power centers. But we have a choice. Every time we choose to listen to the wise and good counsel of the Conscience, every time we choose to serve the *shreya* and sacrifice the *preya*, every time we practice *ahimsa* toward ourselves and others, every time we use the *Bridge of Yoga* to base our outer actions on our inner wisdom, we build our reserves of healing energy, will power and creativity. These are the resources we need to resolve life's seemingly unresolvable challenges. This is how transformative change becomes a reality.

### Establishing a Philosophy of Life

On July 4, 1776, the Declaration of Independence proclaimed that Americans were "free and independent," and "endowed by their Creator with [the] unalienable rights [of] life, liberty and the pursuit of happiness." But merely declaring the belief that we were free in 1776 did not assure that we would live free of pain, misery and bondage today in the 21st century. Clearly, there are serious inequities in our society that must be addressed. And in the end, we must also understand that true freedom is not something that can be given to us by anyone but ourselves.

Unfortunately, in today's world of complex challenges, "freedom" is often reduced to the notion of our ability to come and go as we please, and to choose what we like and discard the rest. But when we habitually over-indulge our personal likes and dislikes, all our relation-ships suffer because happiness becomes dependent on getting everything *my* way.

Real freedom is a very personal matter, and can only be experienced when each of us sincerely invests our time and energy in developing and employing a reliable and meaningful philosophy of life—based on a scientific template of personal experimentation and verification. Without that effort our experience of freedom will remain superficial and sometimes counterproductive, and hu-mankind will continue to exist in perpetual cycles of pleas-ure and pain.

When we thoroughly examine the concept of freedom in the light of our own experiences, we'll begin to under-stand that in every situation *real* freedom means having the liberty to act in ways that will benefit the whole while providing each of us the lasting health, happiness and security we deeply desire.

Yoga Science and Yoga Psychology provide two of the most practical, proven and reliable methods to resolve the challenges of today. They are Self-Reliance and Response-Ability. These practices require the regular employment of our Conscience to access our own inner wisdom, and to choose wisely in the midst of all the powerful influences of family, race, religion, gender, age, work, politics and culture. If we can faithfully do this work, we and everyone on our planet will benefit.

## One Final Thought

As you've learned from reading this short book, Your Conscience is the *only* Function of the Mind that has the power to discriminate, determine, judge and decide. When you understand and employ this Truth, it will become a profoundly positive influence in determining the kind of life you live. This ancient teaching means that *every* decision you have ever made, or will ever make, has and will be made by your Conscience. That's right. Throughout your entire life as a human being, every choice you make is *always* authored by your Conscience. The body itself cannot act unless and until it's empowered by the Conscience. The other Functions of the Mind—the Ego, Senses and Unconscious Mind—possess the power to advise, but *never* to decide. Contemplate that for a moment. Just possessing this knowledge can be your source of tremendous creativity and power in the world!

But here's the rub. Since you, and most of your fellow citizens, were never taught to regularly coordinate all Four Functions of the Mind, the ability of your Conscience to reflect your Super Conscious Wisdom is presently compromised. Consequently, during the mind's decision-making process, the quiet whisper of the Conscience is often overwhelmed by the relatively loud and insistent voices of the Ego, Senses and Unconscious Mind. In that challenging situation, the Conscience will still decide what to do and what not to do (since it's the *only* mind function that has that capacity), but its decisions will be based on limited and possibly faulty input. However, each time you consciously enlist the Conscience to guide your decisions and cultivate the cooperation of the Ego, Senses and Unconscious Mind, you will increasingly gain access to your Inner Wisdom. This is the wisdom that will flawlessly guide your thoughts, words and deeds, preparing you to be skillful in every relationship and circumstance.

The great tragedy of our times is that so many of us do not understand the "why" or the "how" of coordinating the Four Functions of the Mind. This is not a moral failing. It is simply a failure of education. We are neither aware of the enormous value nor the straightforward process of training our mind and living our life guided by the Conscience. As a result, billions of people worldwide unwittingly embrace lifestyle choices that eventually injure health, impair peace of mind, inflict suffering on others, limit possibilities, and eventually threaten the very integrity of society and the Earth—all because we were never trained to use our mind in ways that can profoundly benefit us personally, and humanity as a whole.

Contrast this bleak picture with the quiet revolution that took place in India thousands of years ago. During that time, certain women and men who deeply desired a more rewarding life prayerfully listened to this *Gayatri Mantra* every day: "O, Inner Dweller, Divine Mother, my heart is enveloped in darkness. I pray You will remove the darkness from my vision, and bring the illumination of Supreme Truth by awakening, strengthening and purifying the mind's Conscience so that I can skillfully discriminate between passing pleasure and perennial joy." We would do well to listen to that same mantra today!

To effectively manage the daily avalanche of information you face, and to solve all your urgent challenges, you need only learn to maximize the competence of your most powerful instrument—your mind. When you coordinate all Four Functions of the Mind, the Conscience can reliably reflect your own Super Conscious Wisdom and motivate you to think, speak and act much more creatively than ever before.

With your Conscience as your guide, you can act, not as a limited and habituated individual, but as a vital instrument of the One all-encompassing Supreme Intelligence. You will come to understand your true purpose and begin living each day to fulfill it. And you will immediately begin to discover the creativity and will power that is required to solve all of your challenges. This transformational process is not fiction. It is a practical, scientific, reproducible methodology for attaining the *summum bonum*—the highest and ultimate good—of life.

But please, as I have said many times in these pages, don't believe me. Don't accept on blind faith any advice I've presented in this book. Instead, be motivated enough to turn your own mind-body-sense complex into a scientific laboratory and experiment with what you've learned. *Test* the knowledge I have shared. Only then will you know, and know that you know, that you already have everything you need to create a joyful, creative, healthy and rewarding life. I have every confidence in you.

Namaste.

# *About the Authors*

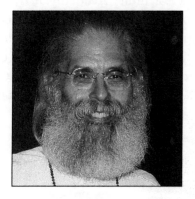

**Leonard Perlmutter**

Leonard (Ram Lev) is the founder and director of The American Meditation Institute in Averill Park, New York, and the originator of National Conscience Month. Leonard is the author and editor of *Transformation—The Journal of Yoga Science as Holistic Mind/Body Medicine,* and over the past decades has served on the faculties of the New England Institute of Ayurvedic Medicine and the International Himalayan Yoga Teachers Association. Leonard has studied in Rishikesh, India and is a direct disciple of Swami Rama of the Himalayas—the man who, in laboratory conditions at the Menninger Institute, demonstrated that blood pressure, heart rate and the autonomic nervous system can be voluntarily controlled. These research demonstrations have been one of the major cornerstones of the modern mind/body movement.

Mr. Perlmutter has presented informative Yoga Science and meditation workshops at the M.D. Anderson Cancer Center, Kaiser Permanente, *The New York Times* Forum on Yoga, the Commonwealth Club of California, the University of Connecticut School of Medicine, the Washington University Medical School, the University of Colorado Medical School, the University of Wisconsin School of Nursing, the U.S. Military Academy at West Point Association of Graduates, the Albany Medical College, and Berkshire Medical Center. Since 2009, Leonard's *Heart and Science of Yoga*® course curriculum has been certified by the Albany Medical College, the American Medical Association and the American Nurses Association for continuing medical education credit.

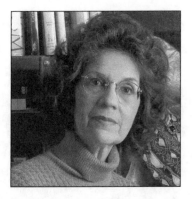

**Jenness Cortez Perlmutter**

Jenness Cortez Perlmutter, co-founder and co-director of the American Meditation Institute, has been a student of Yoga Science since 1973. With her husband, Leonard, she has studied in Rishikesh, India and is a direct disciple of Sri Swami Rama of the Himalayas. Jenness is a graduate of the Herron School of Art and attended the Art Students League of New York. Her acclaimed paintings appear in public, private and corporate collections worldwide.

# The American Meditation Institute
*For Yoga Science and Philosophy*

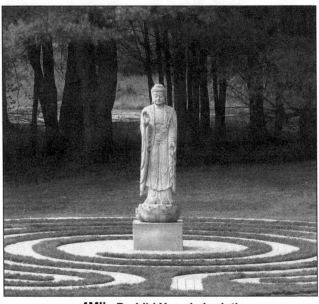

**AMI's Buddhi Yoga Labyrinth**

The American Meditation Institute was established in 1996 for the teaching and practice of authentic Yoga Science and philosophy. Located in the picturesque foothills of the Berkshire Mountains, *AMI* provides a peaceful, healthy setting for learning practical, holistic skills that improve physical, mental, emotional and spiritual well being.

As a living link in the world's oldest, continuous meditation tradition, *AMI* offers a variety of classes (online and at the Home Center in Averill Park, NY) and retreats that:

1. Empower students by awakening them to their individual potentials, freedom of choice and a vision of their own true spiritual nature.

2. Help students embrace those values which have the power to protect, uphold and transform the individual and society.

3. Help students understand and implement these values more completely through the regular, systematic practice of meditation and Yoga Science in their daily lives.

4. Help students recognize and appreciate that these same values are also found within the teachings of their own spiritual traditions.

### Yoga Science and *AMI* Meditation Classes, Summer Retreat and Transformation Journal

Numerous classes (many online), the annual *AMI* summer retreat, and quarterly *Transformation* journal are offered throughout the year. Call, or visit our website for specific details at **americanmeditation.org**

### Membership

The American Meditation Institute is a 501(c)3 non-profit educational organization. Please call, write or visit our website for information on how you can support this teaching.

### Speaker's Bureau

If you or your school, church, temple, mosque, yoga center, government, business, or civic organization is interested in hosting a workshop by Leonard Perlmutter, please contact The American Meditation Institute to make arrangements.

### How to Contact *AMI*

For further information about our programs, please contact us at Tel. (518) 674-8714, 60 Garner Road, Averill Park, NY 12018, email: **info@americanmeditation.org**.

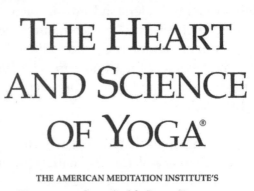
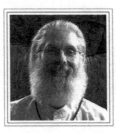

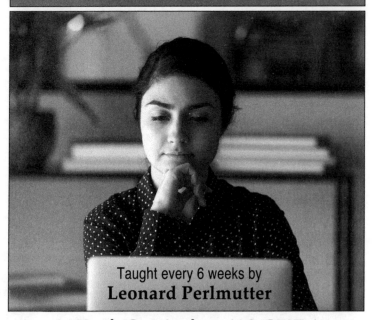

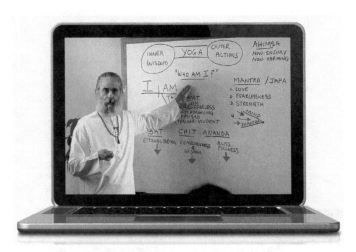

## *The Perfect Video Companion To*
# THE HEART AND SCIENCE OF YOGA®

Containing all the Core Curriculum in 40 convenient lecture segments

Meditation • Mantra Science • Diaphragmatic Breathing • Yoga Psychology • Easy-Gentle Yoga
Life After Death • Mind Function Optimization • Lymph System Detox • Nutrition • Ayurvedic Medicine • Prayer

### 5 1/2 Hour Online Video Course
## Comprehensive Meditation & Easy-Gentle Yoga
### WITH LEONARD PERLMUTTER

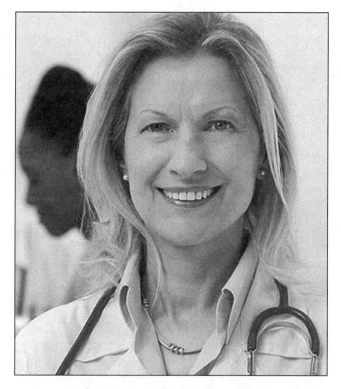

*The American Meditation Institute Offers*
**Classes and Conferences for
Physicians and other Healthcare Providers**

## THE HEART AND SCIENCE OF YOGA®

Comprehensive Training in Yoga Science as

# Holistic Mind/Body Medicine

A Unique Continuing Medical Education Curriculum Developed for
Clinical Application • Personal Health
Relieving Physician Burnout and Building Resilience

## with Leonard Perlmutter (Ram Lev)

**For current dates and information**
**info@americanmeditation.org    Tel. (518) 674-8714**

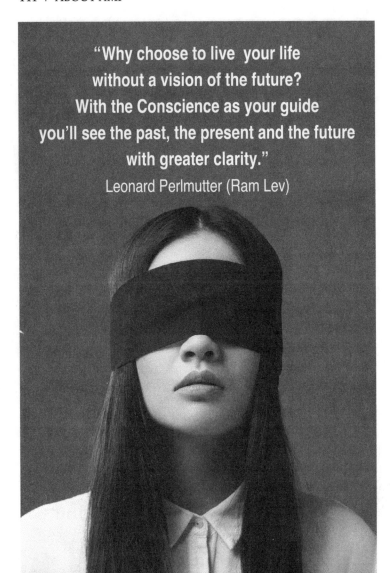